"At last, a thorough, accurate, and up-to-date book on breast reconstruction. It's long overdue for women facing the confusing choices after mastectomy."

Dean Edell, MD

"An important and much needed book covered in a comprehensive and easily-understood manner."

Patricia T. Kelly, PhD
Medical Geneticist

"This book is a must. It is what women need in today's complicated medical world."

Michael O'Holleran, MD

"Even with today's heightened awareness of breast cancer, there are still many myths and misunderstandings relating to breast reconstruction. The most important thing a patient can do is to educate herself on her options so she can be an active part of her treatment team. A resource such as *The Breast Reconstruction Guidebook,* which provides a compilation of information, is of great value to patients."

Frederic J. Duffy, Jr., MD, FACS

"At a time when they're most vulnerable, women who lose their breasts to cancer must make decisions that will impact them for the rest of their lives, often without the information they need. Finally, women have a blueprint of the reconstruction process. They have choices. This book explains them all."

Sue Friedman, Executive Director
FORCE: Facing Our Risk of Cancer Empowered

"*The Breast Reconstruction Guidebook* acts as a well-informed friend. It answers many of the big (and little) questions women have as they cope with the physical and emotional turmoil of breast cancer."

Claudia Pratt, RN, MA, BSN, Nurse Coordinator
Seton Breast Health Center

"If you are a woman who has been diagnosed with breast cancer and will be treated with a mastectomy, *The Breast Reconstruction Guidebook* is the book to read. It is a worthwhile guide to wholeness and satisfaction."

Brenda Gill, Hotline Peer Counselor
Y-ME National Breast Cancer Organization

The Breast Reconstruction Guidebook

Issues and Answers
from Research to Recovery

by
Kathy Steligo

With a foreward by
Gail Lebovic, MA, MD, FACS
Clinical Assistant Professor of Surgery
Stanford Medical Center

Carlo Press
San Carlos, CA

This book is not intended as a substitute for medical advice. It is sold with the understanding that neither the author nor publisher is engaged in rendering medical or other professional advice. Consult your physician before adopting the suggestions in this book.

Cover and interior design: Fischer Design

Publisher's Cataloging-in-Publication

Steligo, Kathy
    The Breast Reconstruction Guidebook: Issues and Answers from Research to Recovery / Kathy Steligo

     p. cm.

Includes index.
ISBN: 0-9669799-6-6
LCCN: 2003107244

1. Breast Cancer 2. Mastectomy 3. Breast Reconstruction

RC280.B8S 2003

616.99'449—dc21

Printed and bound in the United States of America.

Contact the publisher about quantity discounts for your company, school or health organization.

For Charles: you were right, we did get through it.

For every woman who faces mastectomy and reconstruction: you will get through it too.

Acknowledgements

To Dr. Gail Lebovic, thank you on so many levels, for your surgical skill, humor, hugs, text review, and the photos. You're the best.

To Dr. Fred Marcus, I couldn't possibly write a book related to breast cancer without thanking my oncologist. Although you weren't involved directly in my reconstruction, I'm grateful for your compassion, insight, and expertise.

To Sue Friedman, Executive Director, FORCE: Facing Our Risk of Cancer Empowered, my sincerest gratitude for reviewing and improving the manuscript.

To more than 400 women who graciously answered my interview questions and shared their personal reconstruction experiences, I thank you on behalf of every one who reads this book. Your words help make the story real.

To countless nurses, doctors, and other medical professionals who took time from their hectic schedules to answer my questions and clarify issues, a very big thank you.

Author's note: Thousands of skilled and dedicated reconstructive surgeons are committed to restoring women's breasts and self-image after mastectomy. Some of these wonderful surgeons are men; some are women. For the sake of simplicity, surgeons are referred to as "he" throughout the text.

Credits

A very big thank you to the following for providing illustrations and photographs.

American Cancer Society, Inc.: *Exercises after Breast Surgery* (p. 159-166), reprinted by permission.

Breastcancer.org, a nonprofit organization dedicated to providing the most reliable, complete, and up-to-date information about breast cancer: cells (p. 7), TRAM flap (p. 94).

Coloplast Breast Care: prostheses (p. 14).

Dr. Frederick J. Duffy, Jr.: perforator flap (p. 92).

Dr. Daryl K. Hoffman: patient photos (p. 95).

Dr. Gail Lebovic: patient photos (ch. 2, 9, 13, 14).

Fischer Design: upper torso (p. 25, 119), decision roadmap (p. 57), expansion (p.85), abdomen (p. 93), gluteal flap (p. 109), breast reduction (p. 116), star flap (p. 124), surgical drain (p. 152).

Inamed Aesthetics: breast anatomy (p. 5), mastectomy and delayed reconstruction (p. 26, 74), implants (p. 70), patient photos (p. 87).

Permark: tattoo color chart (p. 125).

F. W. Evans: woman-front and back views (p. 90, 105).

Contents

Decision: Mastectomy

Anatomy of the breast
A breast cancer primer
Surgical treatments
Do you really need a mastectomy?

Empty chest
The prosthesis alternative
Breast reconstruction

Sorting through the options
Matching the opposite breast
Choosing or refusing

The mastectomy procedure
Immediate reconstruction
Delayed reconstruction
Coordinating reconstruction with adjuvant therapies

Finding Answers, Making Decisions

Reconstructive Procedures

Recovery
Are implants right for you?
Potential problems

10. The Expander Experience .84

Getting your fill
Living in limbo
Exchange surgery
Potential problems

11. Tummy Tuck Flaps 90

Tissue flap basics
The attached TRAM flap
The free TRAM
The DIEP flap
Building a new belly button
Is a TRAM or DIEP right for you?
Comparing abdominal flaps and implants

12. Other Flap Methods 105

The back flap
Gluteal flaps
The thigh flap

13. Altering the Opposite Breast 111

Breast augmentation
Breast reduction
Breast lift

14. Final Touches: Creating the Nipple and Areola 121

Icing on the cake
Building the nipple
Adding the areola
Problems and solutions
Non-Surgical alternatives

From Prep to Post-Op

Recovery and Beyond

Foreward

Breast cancer strikes fear in each and every one of us. The thought of losing one or both breasts is every woman's nightmare. Luckily, we are winning the fight. Mammograms find at least 50 percent of all breast cancers in the United States before they can be felt by examination. Although more and more women are candidates for breast conservation therapy, for some, removing the breast tissue is the only choice, or is the optimal method of treatment.

Major strides have been made in the many ways to reconstruct the breast. In most cases, the process begins immediately at the time of mastectomy. Researching and learning subtle differences between the many options, however, is truly an overwhelming task for most women and their families when they are dealing with a diagnosis of cancer.

This masterful book by Kathy Steligo promises to be the ultimate guide to reconstruction for patients, family, and friends. In a straightforward and easy to read fashion, she lays out the details of each reconstructive technique. This invaluable text will no doubt become an essential tool for anyone touched by this disease. If you, or someone you care about has breast cancer, give them the gift of your loving support and a copy of this book. You can read it all in one night. I did!

Best wishes for good health.

Gail S. Lebovic, MA, MD, FACS
Clinical Assistant Professor of Surgery
Stanford Medical Hospital

Introduction

Many cancer patients say their disease is a learning experience. That's certainly been the case with my own breast cancer. I've heard those four horrible words—"you have breast cancer"—three times, had four biopsies, two lumpectomies, eight weeks of radiation, a sentinel node biopsy, genetic counseling, genetic testing, bilateral mastectomies and reconstruction with saline implants. While I would never have chosen these particular opportunities for learning, each one, in its own way, has given me more insight into the disease, into myself, and compassion for other women who lose their breasts.

When I went looking for reconstructive options, I hoped to find a book like this. I found plenty of books on breast cancer. Some provided a cursory chapter or two about reconstruction, but none had the comprehensive information I needed. I wanted an objective, single source that didn't favor one technique over the other; something that translated the technical terms and procedures into understandable concepts, and explained the practical aspects of recovery and life after mastectomy. That single source didn't exist. And that's why I wrote this book—to share what I've learned with you and other women who wonder what reconstruction is really like.

To my own mountain of research, I added information from clinical studies and medical journals, and perspectives from oncologists, surgeons, nurses, and other medical professionals. More than 400 women took the time to share their own experiences and offer information they wished they had before reconstruction; many of their comments are included.

Mastectomy is a shocking pronouncement. Your doctor may recommend it to eliminate your breast cancer (who knew that "catching it early" might also mean losing a breast?). Perhaps you've decided it's the best way to reduce your risk of developing the disease. Maybe you're trying to decide between lumpectomy with radiation or mastectomy. Whatever your circumstances, you have alternatives after losing your breast. These choices require decisions. Decisions require information.

You won't find answers in this book, but you will find the information you need to make your own decisions. You may decide reconstruction is right for you. You may not. Either way, you'll understand the benefits and limitations of each reconstructive technique, and what to expect each step of the way: before your surgery, in the hospital, during recovery, and life beyond reconstruction.

The Boy Scouts are right. It's good to be prepared. Get comfy in your favorite chair. Highlight paragraphs that particularly appeal so you can find them easily when you need them. Take it all in and give yourself time to absorb what you read. Take control of your choices. Enjoy a healthy, confident, and happy future.

Decision: Mastectomy

Chapter 1

Why Mastectomy?

No coward soul is mine.
No trembler in the world's storm-troubled sphere;
I see Heaven's glories shine,
and faith shines, arming me from fear.

– Emily Bronte

"You have breast cancer."

Do any other four words hold greater fear for women? Your stomach falls and your heart seems to stop as your brain struggles to make sense of the words. You're sure your report was mixed up with some other poor soul's, and you wonder if you'll die. Your doctor says he has good news: you'll live—but one or both of your breasts must be removed. For many women, this trade-off is as devastating as the diagnosis itself.

Put in perspective, what woman wouldn't choose her life over her breasts? Still, losing one or both breasts can dent even the strongest woman's sense of well-being and self image. Losing any part of the body is a personal affront, let alone one so uniquely feminine. As young girls, we're impatient for our budding breasts to grow. As mature women, our breasts are physically and emotionally significant: they define much of our physical profiles, provide pleasure, and feed our babies. We're fearful and saddened when cancer takes that away.

Breast cancer is an insidious disease. One day you're healthy, the next day your breast is gone. In the United States, more than 100,000 women have mastectomies annually. Each woman has her own concerns: Will mastectomy eliminate her cancer? How will she look afterward? In most situations, removing breast tissue does eliminate breast cancer. Afterward, talented plastic surgeons using sophisticated reconstructive techniques can create new breasts with implants or a woman's own tissue.

Like most things in life, reconstruction has benefits and limitations. To appreciate both, we must first understand breast cancer and mastectomy. To do that, it makes sense to start at the beginning: the breast.

Anatomy of the Breast

Breasts are essentially big glands designed to make milk. Positioned over the *pectoralis major* and *pectoralis minor* chest muscles, breasts are surrounded by tissue and fat and bound together by skin. They contain no muscle—that's why no amount of exercise can make them bigger.

In our 20s and 30s, our breasts are more dense tissue than fat. This tissue makes the youthful breast firm. It's also the reason mammograms aren't routinely recommended for women under 40, because dense tissue and abnormalities look alike on film. As women's health expert Dr. Susan Love says, "It's like looking for a polar bear in the snow." As we age—particularly after menopause—much of our breast tissue is replaced by fat, and our once-firm breasts begin to sag. Not so great for our profiles, but very good for mammograms, because fat stands out in contrast to abnormalities.

Most breast cancers begin in the *lobules* or *ducts*. Lobules produce breast milk; ducts deliver it to the nipple.

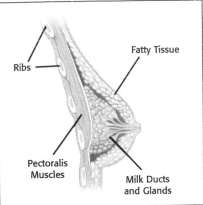

Ribs

Fatty Tissue

Pectoralis Muscles

Milk Ducts and Glands

The breast is made of fatty tissue, lobules, and ducts surrounded by skin. Throughout the breast and nipple, a network of nerves reacts to heat, cold, touch and other sensations.

The lymph system. The body's immune system includes little bean-shaped *lymph nodes* under the arm. The nodes collect, filter, and recycle breast fluids and cellular waste drained from the breast. They also trap bacteria and cancerous cells. That's why lymph nodes are removed and examined whenever invasive breast cancer is diagnosed—to determine whether the cancer has spread beyond the breast to the lymph system, or *metastasized*, migrated to other parts of the body. Some or all of the nodes may be removed, depending on the nature of the cancer. Unfortunately, this *axillary node dissection* sometimes impairs the lymph system. Fluids may back up in the arm, causing *lymphedema*, a mild-to-severe swelling that can occur weeks, months, or even years after surgery. Chapter 19 describes how to discourage and manage lymphedema.

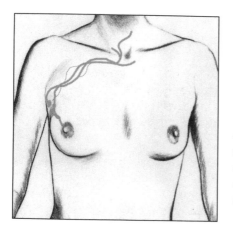

The underarm lymph system collects and filters most breast fluids. Secondary lymph systems are located above the collarbone and under the ribcage near the breastbone.

Sentinel node biopsy. Axillary node dissection has long been a standard diagnostic procedure for invasive cancers. Now surgeons can perform a *sentinel node biopsy*, a less invasive technique, for women with early-stage breast cancer. If cancer has spread beyond the breast, the sentinel node is most likely to contain the destructive cells. This new technique is effective and reduces the risk of lymphedema. It can be done as an outpatient procedure with a local anesthesia, or under general anesthesia with lumpectomy or mastectomy.

The surgeon injects blue dye and/or a radioactive liquid into the tumor site. In about an hour, these materials drain from the breast to the sentinel node. By using a mini-Geiger counter or following the path of the blue dye, the surgeon can identify and remove the sentinel node. If the node is free of cancer cells, the rest of the body is likely to be clear as well, and the remaining nodes are spared. If the node is positive for cancerous cells, an axillary dissection is performed to determine the extent of the cancer and appropriate treatment.

Your urine may be blue for a day or two after a sentinel node biopsy. It may take six to 12 months for the dye to fade completely from your breast. Ask your surgeon if you're a candidate for a sentinel node biopsy, and if he's experienced with the procedure.

A Breast Cancer Primer

We all dread the "C" word. But what, exactly, is cancer? It occurs when environmental, lifestyle, or hereditary factors cause cells—in this case, breast cells—to mutate and grow uncontrollably. Cancer cells are rogues. They multiply and lump together, forming cancerous tumors.

Breast cancer grows for an average of six to eight years before it can be detected by a mammogram. It takes about 10 years before a lump can be felt. If you find a lump in your breast or mammography detects a questionable spot, the first step is to biopsy the site by removing a small tissue sample. This is done surgically or with a special needle and then sent to a pathologist, who determines whether breast cancer is present. If it is, he identifies and classifies the cancer to help your doctor determine a course of treatment. Eighty percent of biopsies prove to be *benign* or non-cancerous.

Non-invasive breast cancers are said to be *in situ*, or "in place," because they remain within the confines of the lobules or ducts. Other *invasive* or *infiltrating* cancers are more worrisome, because they can spread to the breast tissue or other areas of the body. Seen under a microscope, breast cancer cells look like this:

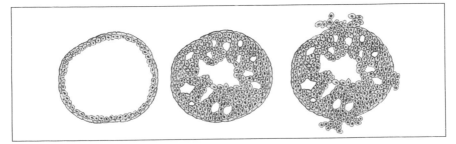

Normal, healthy cells (left), non-invasive cancer cells (center), and invasive cancer cells (right).

Non-invasive breast cancers. *Ductal carcinoma in situ (DCIS)* is the most common non-invasive breast cancer. It is an early-stage cancer contained within the ducts. Almost all cases are found by mammography. Virtually all women diagnosed with DCIS are completely cured.

Lobular carcinoma in situ (LCIS). This cancer begins in the lobules of the breast. Although it isn't a true cancer, women with LCIS are monitored carefully, because they are at higher risk of developing invasive breast cancer.

Invasive breast cancers. About 80 percent of all breast cancers diagnosed have the ability to spread beyond the breast. *Invasive* or *infiltrating ductal carcinoma (IDC)* begins in the ducts and spreads to the breast tissue. IDC accounts for most invasive breast cancers.

Invasive or *infiltrating lobular carcinoma* (ILC). Hard to detect, ILC is similar to IDC, except it begins in the lobules rather than the ducts. Only 10 percent of invasive breast cancers are ILC.

Paget's Disease. This rare breast cancer begins in the ducts and spreads to the nipple and areola. It may occur with either invasive or non-invasive breast cancers.

Inflammatory breast cancer. This very aggressive, uncommon invasive cancer affects the breast skin. Symptoms include a very hard breast, or skin that is warm, red, swollen, or develops little pockmarks resembling the skin of an orange.

Breast Cancer Facts

- The leading cancer in women.
- The second leading cause of cancer deaths in women (after lung cancer).
- Most women do not die from breast cancer. Millions of survivors are thriving around the world.
- 80 percent of breast lumps are not cancerous.

Estimated new cases in 2003 (invasive):   211,300

Estimated new cases in 2003 (non-invasive):   55,700

Estimated deaths in 2003:   39,800

Source: American Cancer Society

Surgical Treatments

Before the era of early detection began in the mid-1980s, breast tumors were usually quite large by the time they were discovered. Almost all women diagnosed with breast cancer were treated alike, with little regard for individual condition or personal choice. A woman entering the hospital for a biopsy didn't know whether she would wake up with or without her breasts. If cancer was found, her breast, lymph nodes, and underlying chest muscle were removed. No questions, no getting used to the idea, and no alternatives.

Thankfully, those days are behind us. We're living in an age of patient participation. Breast conservation, when prudent, is the treatment of choice. When conservative methods cannot effectively eliminate cancer, improved mastectomy procedures allow for faster healing and a variety of reconstructive options. Mastectomy is surgical removal of the entire breast:

Unilateral mastectomy is removal of one breast.

Bilateral mastectomy is removal of both breasts.

Prophylactic mastectomy is removal of healthy breasts to reduce a woman's risk of developing breast cancer.

Breast-conserving surgeries. Women with a single, small incidence of DCIS or early-stage tumors without positive nodes can choose *lumpectomy*—removal of the tumor and some of the surrounding tissue—and radiation. A small scar remains from the incision. Although the shape and size of the breast may change somewhat, reconstruction isn't usually necessary. Women who have lumpectomy and radiation have the same rate of survival as women with mastectomies, but a somewhat higher rate of recurrence.

When a larger tumor is involved, a *quadrantectomy* may be appropriate. A larger segment of tissue, skin, and the lining of the chest muscle are removed. The nipple remains, except in the case of Paget's Disease, or when the tumor is located directly under the nipple. Breast shape can be restored by rearranging the remaining tissue (reducing the overall size of the breast). Like lumpectomy, quadrantectomy is usually followed by radiation.

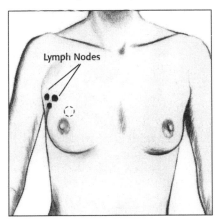

A lumpectomy removes a small tumor and some of the surrounding tissue. Some lymph nodes may also be removed.

Mastectomy is recommended when lumpectomy or quadrantectomy can't effectively treat breast cancer, as in the following conditions:

- Cancer is found in two or more areas of the breast.

- The breast or chest has been previously irradiated.

- The cancerous area extends beyond the edges of the biopsy.

- Removing a large tumor from a small breast would be disfiguring.

- The patient has lupus, other connective tissue disorders, or health conditions that preclude her from having radiation.

Mastectomies. A *total mastectomy* removes the breast tissue, nipple, areola, and some skin around the incision. This surgery is commonly used to treat DCIS in two or more areas of the breast, or when the cancerous area extends beyond the edges of the biopsy. No lymph nodes are removed.

A *modified radical mastectomy* is similar to a total mastectomy but includes either axillary dissection or sentinel node biopsy. This is now the most commonly performed mastectomy.

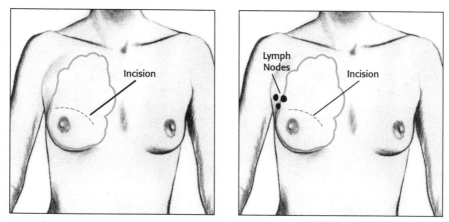

A total mastectomy (left) removes the breast tissue and skin. A modified radical mastectomy (right) also removes some or all lymph nodes under the arm.

The *radical (Halsted) mastectomy* was standard treatment for breast cancer until the 1970s. This was a very disfiguring procedure, because it removed the chest muscle, lymph nodes, and skin along with the breast. Patients were left with a concave chest, considerable pain, and a high risk of lymphedema. Radical mastectomy is now rarely necessary.

Do You Really Need a Mastectomy?

Why is mastectomy recommended for some women and not for others? Treatment is defined by how far the cancer has spread, its aggressive nature, and the woman's risk of recurrence. The more aggressive the cancer, the more aggressive the treatment. In some cases, women have a choice between lumpectomy with radiation or mastectomy.

American women with breast cancer are more likely to have mastectomy than women in other developed countries. According to one study of 9,000 women with early-stage cancers, women in the United States have mastectomies 43 percent more often than their counterparts in Britain.

Although lumpectomy with radiation is as effective as mastectomy in treating early-stage cancer, about one-third of women who are eligible choose mastectomy instead. A 1999 study at a New Hampshire hospital asked 40 surgeons (26 men and 14 women) to imagine they were women with early-stage breast cancer. They were told to choose a treatment for themselves, assuming lumpectomy with radiation or mastectomy was equally effective. Half chose mastectomy. The results were identical for both male and female surgeons.

It was bothersome going to the hospital every day for radiation, but it was worth it to keep my breast. – Lola

My friend's breast shriveled to almost nothing after radiation. I preferred to have a mastectomy. – Ynez

If your physician recommends mastectomy, get a second opinion from a doctor in a different medical group. Better yet, get two second opinions: one on your diagnosis, another on the need for mastectomy. Send your medical history, mammogram, pathology slides, and reports to the best breast center, teaching university, or specialist in the country, no matter what the initial diagnosis.

Only you can make the decision whether mastectomy or lumpectomy with radiation is right for you. Taking a couple of weeks to get a second opinion will be well worth your time. You have nothing to lose, and it just might save your breast. If you decide mastectomy is your best course of action, you have choices about how you'll look after your breast is removed.

Chapter 2

Post-Mastectomy Options

If you can talk, you can sing.
If you can walk, you can dance.

– Ancient saying from Zimbabwe

If mastectomy is the best treatment choice for you, you have an important decision to make. What will you do about your missing breast? You have three options to consider.

Empty Chest

Years ago, a flat chest was a woman's only alternative after mastectomy. For some, it's still the option of choice. Many women simply don't feel the need to replace their breasts. Some small-breasted women, for example, don't consider mastectomy a significant change. Others feel radically changed by their cancer experience. They embrace their flat chests as a way of acknowledging mastectomy and their post-cancer personas.

If you have bilateral mastectomies, both sides of your chest will be flat. A unilateral mastectomy, however, presents a practical problem. Because one breast is missing and one remains, you may feel unbalanced or lopsided and find it difficult to fit into some clothes. If you wear a bra or bathing suit, one side will be empty.

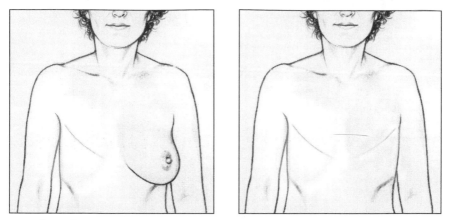

A unilateral mastectomy leaves one side of your chest flat (left). Both sides are flat after a bilateral mastectomy (right).

The Prosthesis Alternative

A *prosthesis* is an artificial breast form worn to give the appearance of a natural breast. (Prosthesis is singular; *prostheses* is plural.) A well-made prosthesis provides balance with your healthy breast and creates a natural shape under clothing. If you're undecided about rebuilding your breast, or you must delay reconstruction due to chemotherapy or radiation treatment, you can use a prosthesis during the in-between interval.

Breast forms are available in a variety of sizes, shapes, and skin tones. Some are positioned on the chest with adhesive and can be worn without a bra. Others fit into special pockets sewn into bras, bathing suits, and other garments. You can even buy artificial nipples to apply to your breast form; more expensive models have built-in nipples. Comfort and feel vary greatly, depending on the materials used. Cost runs from $15 for the least expensive to $2,500 for custom-made forms.

- Cotton prostheses fill a bra cup, but have no natural breast qualities. Although soft and comfortable, these inexpensive forms provide the least shape. From $15.

- Polyfill or foam breast forms are often used as "starter" prostheses after mastectomy, until you've healed sufficiently to wear a heavier, more permanent form. If you call Reach to Recovery (800-227-2345) several weeks before your mastectomy, a volunteer will bring a temporary prostheses and a mastectomy bra to the hospital and show you how to use them. From $25.

- Rubber or latex forms look better than cotton, polyfill, or foam prostheses, but often feel rubbery and don't have the weight or natural feel of silicone. From $25.

- Silicone prostheses move and feel like a natural breast. Available in a variety of shades to match skin tone, silicone forms are the most expensive, but you get what you pay for. From $150 to $500.

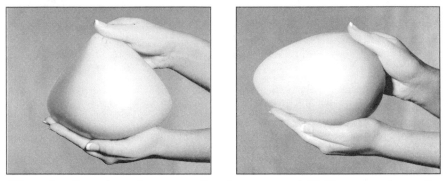

Triangular shaped prostheses are sloped at the top (left). The tapered end of a teardrop shaped form (right) provides a better fit when more tissue is lost from the underarm or upper chest.

Where to shop. Nordstrom, Sears, Land's End, JC Penney, and many other department stores sell prostheses in their lingerie departments. Small specialty shops that cater to post-mastectomy patients are often listed in the phone directory under "Mastectomy Forms & Supplies" or "Prosthetics." The American Cancer Society (ACS) offers a good selection of reasonably priced prostheses and mastectomy products in its TLC catalog (800-850-9445 or www.tlccatalog.org). Prostheses are also available on the Internet. Getting an exact fit can be an issue, however, if you can't try on a prostheses before you buy it.

Tips for Buying Prostheses

- Let a qualified fitter help you find the right size prostheses.
- Take someone with you so you'll have a second opinion about how you look with different types of prostheses.
- If you've had a unilateral mastectomy, it's important to match the weight and size of your healthy breast.
- If you prefer a prosthesis that sticks to your chest, ask for a sample of the adhesive before you buy, so you can make sure it doesn't cause an allergic reaction.
- Consider prostheses of different weights and fabrics for different purposes or occasions.

Paying for Your Prostheses. The Women's Health and Cancer Rights Act (WHCRA) of 1998 requires insurance companies who pay for mastectomy to also cover either reconstruction or prostheses. Insurers are not required to pay for both. If you put in a claim for a prosthesis after your mastectomy, then later decide to have reconstruction, your insurance may not pay for your surgery.

If your doctor provides a prescription, most health insurance companies will pay for a new prosthesis every two years and two special bras each year. If you don't have insurance coverage and can't afford a prosthesis, contact your local ACS chapter or the Y-ME National Breast Cancer Organization (800-221-2141 or www.y-me.org). Both organizations provide free prostheses and special bras to women of limited income.

Breast Reconstruction

Surgical reconstruction is the process of repairing physical defects caused by injury, trauma, or disease. Talented plastic surgeons can rebuild facial features, skulls, arms, hands, and feet. They can also create breasts after mastectomy, with the techniques described in Chapters 9-14. Reconstruction is more complex and requires more surgical skill than *breast augmentation*, which uses implants to increase the size of healthy breasts.

A general surgeon performs your breast biopsy, lumpectomy, and mastectomy. A plastic surgeon or specially trained breast surgeon performs reconstruction. The "plastic" in plastic surgery, by the way, refers to *plastikos*, a Greek word meaning "to form" or "to mold."

Reconstruction can't give you a perfect breast, but it can soften the harshness of mastectomy and help restore your feeling of physical wholeness. Reconstruction is also a more acceptable solution for women who don't want to be bothered with putting on and taking off prostheses. With your physical symmetry restored, you can wear the same clothing you wore before mastectomy, including lingerie and bathing suits, without special bras or prostheses. You'll be the only one who knows you have a reconstructed breast.

A growing demand. According to the American Society of Plastic Surgeons (ASPS), breast reconstruction is now the sixth most-often performed reconstructive procedure in North America. The organization's member surgeons performed almost 82,000 breast reconstructions in 2001.

Top Six Reconstructive Procedures (1992-2001)			
PROCEDURE	1992	2001	PERCENT INCREASE
Tumor Removal	502,567	4,051,071	706
Laceration repair	135,494	441,917	226
Hand surgery	138,233	235,474	70
Scar revision	52,647	227,911	333
Breast reduction	39,639	99,428	151
Breast reconstruction	29,607	81,729	176

Source: ASPS

An increase of 176 percent in a single decade can be traced to at least five factors:

1. Improved screening methods find more breast cancers.

2. Conservative mastectomies allow for very good reconstructions.

3. Women have several reconstructive choices.

4. Information about reconstruction is more readily available.

5. Federal law requires insurance companies to pay for reconstruction (if the insurer already covers mastectomy).

If you're facing a mastectomy, consider your post-operative alternatives. Weigh the advantages and disadvantages of each option to determine which is best for you.

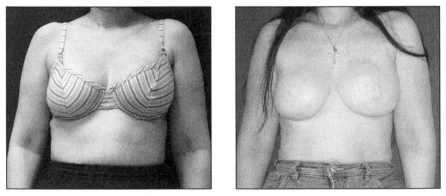

Reconstruction can restore a woman's natural profile in or out of clothes.

Chapter 3

Breast Reconstruction Basics

*Don't let the present overwhelm your sense
of the possibilities of the future.*

– Timothy Forbes

Someday, we'll control breast cancer. We'll know how to prevent it or turn it off, and mastectomy will become obsolete. Until then, reconstruction is our best antidote to losing a breast. Using surgical techniques vastly improved in the last decade, surgeons can now recreate breasts, complete with nipple and areola (the darker area around the nipple). Perhaps the most amazing aspect of reconstruction is the ability to customize breasts to women's individual preferences. Small, large, round, high, droopy—we all have different breast shapes and sizes. Good reconstruction can recreate them all.

Sorting Through the Options

No matter how your breast is rebuilt, it's never a one-step process. Procedures may include two or more operations over several months. The initial surgery forms the breast *mound*—a breast without a nipple or areola. This first stage is the most complex and involves the most recovery. Depending on the procedure you choose, you may need additional surgeries to complete your reconstruction, correct problems, or refine the breast shape or size. A final optional procedure adds a new nipple and areola.

Implants. About half of all reconstructions involve implants. This surgery is the simplest and least invasive, but the entire reconstruction process stretches over several months. In most cases, a temporary implant called an *expander* is placed under the chest muscle and slowly inflated over several weeks. During a second exchange surgery, the expander is replaced with an implant. Some women have enough skin to cover an implant and don't need the expansion process. Implants are a good reconstructive choice for women who:

- Don't have enough spare tissue to create a breast.

- Don't want additional scarring elsewhere on their body.

- Will have bilateral reconstruction and won't need to match the remaining breast.

- Can't endure a longer operation because of age or health.

Implants and expanders are described in detail in Chapters 9 and 10.

Tissue flaps. Fat and skin from your abdomen, back, or buttocks can make a very natural-looking breast. These tissue transfers or *flaps* are transferred to the chest and shaped into a breast. Unlike implants, flaps form a full-size breast during the initial operation. You go into the operating room with your natural breast and come out with a reconstructed breast in its place. Additional surgery is later performed to refine the breast shape and size and create a nipple. Compared to implants, tissue flaps are more complex and require greater surgical skill. Recovery is more intense, but the overall reconstruction timeline is shorter. Flaps are better options for women who:

- Want a reconstructed breast that looks and feels the most natural.

- Have had previous radiation at the mastectomy site.

- Are willing to accept more scarring compared to implants.

- Don't want to spend several months dealing with expanders.

Flaps are described in detail in Chapters 11 and 12.

Comparing options. The University of Michigan Breast Reconstruction Outcome Survey (MBROS) questioned 397 mastectomy patients to determine their overall satisfaction with reconstruction. The women were surveyed a few days prior to their reconstruction surgery and again a year later. While tissue flap patients were more satisfied overall than implant patients, the study found significant psychological and functional gains in reconstruction patients one year after surgery, regardless of the reconstructive technique.

Women showed improved mental health, emotional well-being, energy level, and satisfaction with the way their breasts looked.

Comparing Reconstructive Techniques

	EXPANDERS/IMPLANTS	TISSUE FLAPS
Surgery	Two short operations 3-6 months apart.	One longer initial procedure.
Anesthesia	General.	General.
Hospital stay	2-3 days when done with mastectomy. Overnight if performed as a separate surgery.	4-7 days whether performed with mastectomy or as separate surgery.
Nipple	Created in a separate procedure.	Created in a separate procedure.
Scars	At mastectomy site.	At mastectomy and donor sites.
Opposite breast	Often requires surgery to achieve symmetry.	Easier to match reconstructed breast without surgery. Opposite breast can also be surgically modified.

Matching the Opposite Breast

If you're going to have unilateral reconstruction, you'll want your new breast to match your natural breast as much as possible. You have three options for achieving symmetry:

Do nothing to the opposite breast. For some women, scarring a healthy breast is an unacceptable choice. If you prefer not to alter your remaining breast in any way, it's easier to match the shape and natural droop with a tissue flap than an implant. Some women can achieve acceptable symmetry without any changes to their opposite breast.

Surgically alter the opposite breast. Your healthy breast can be reduced, enlarged, or lifted during your reconstruction. These procedures are described in Chapter 13.

Remove and reconstruct the opposite breast. If you're at increased risk for breast cancer, you may want to consider prophylactic removal of your healthy breast. In that case, you'll have bilateral mastectomies and reconstruction, and

Breast Reconstruction by Age

AGE	PERCENT OF BREAST RECONSTRUCTION SURGERIES
19-34	5
35-50	51
51-64	36
65 and over	7

Source: ASPS member surgeons (year 2000)

both breasts can be reconstructed at the same time. Prophylactic mastectomy is discussed in Chapter 5.

Choosing or Refusing

Most women can have reconstruction, whether it's performed at the same time as mastectomy or years later. It doesn't matter when the breast is removed or how it looked before. Nor is age a factor, as long as the woman is in good health. Women from 20 to 70-something have had successful reconstruction.

What other women say. When it comes to reconstruction, there is no right or wrong answer. There are only personal decisions. For many women, reconstruction is a no-brainer. For others, it's a confusing and stressful choice. While 75 percent of women have reconstruction after mastectomy, it's not right for everyone. In either case, it pays to thoroughly research your options and know what to expect before you decide whether it is the right procedure for you. If you decide to have reconstruction, you'll have other decisions to make, as you'll discover in Chapter 7.

Women say they choose reconstruction because it:

- Makes them feel whole again.

- Restores confidence in their physical appearance.

- Gives them a sense of control they didn't have with their treatment.

- Isn't a constant reminder of their mastectomy, as is a flat chest or prosthesis.

- Brings a sense of closure to the physical and emotional struggle of breast cancer diagnosis and treatment.

Women who decide against reconstruction say they do so because they:

- Are comfortable without breasts.

- Don't want breasts that have no feeling or aren't "real."

- Don't want to go through additional surgeries and recovery.

- Want to try wearing a prosthesis before committing to more surgery.

- Fear the possibility of surgical complications or unsatisfactory results.

Health concerns. Reconstruction is not particularly dangerous, but there is risk with any surgery. Although uncommon, infection, excessive bleeding, slow-healing wounds, or other problems can occur. Your doctor may advise against reconstructive surgery if you are elderly, frail, or have any of the following conditions:

■ Heart or lung disease, recent stroke, Alzheimer's, advanced diabetes, or chronic high blood pressure.

■ Lupus, scleroderma, or other autoimmune diseases that can weaken your body's ability to fight off infection. Consult with your rheumatologist and surgeon before proceeding with reconstruction.

■ Obesity puts you at higher risk for blood clots, pneumonia, and adverse reactions to anesthesia.

■ Smoking before or after reconstruction surgery increases the chance of infection, constricts the blood flow, and may cause excessive scarring and poor healing.

At 31, I couldn't deal with having no breasts. If I had to have mastectomies, I wanted to restore my breasts as closely as possible, and that meant reconstruction. – Riley

Initially, I thought a prosthesis would be fine under my clothes. I changed my mind about a year after my mastectomy; I guess I was open to a more permanent alternative. – Shelly

Studies by M.D. Anderson Cancer Center, the Cleveland Clinic Foundation, and other health organizations confirm women who smoke have higher rates of post-surgery infection. They are also more likely to experience *necrosis*, or skin death, at both the mastectomy and donor sites. This means the skin around the incision dies due to insufficient blood supply. Women who stop smoking at least three to four weeks before surgery and three to four weeks after surgery seem to fare as well as non-smokers.

Chapter 4

How Mastectomy Affects Reconstruction

If your head tells you one thing and your heart tells you another, before you do anything, you should first decide whether you have a better head or a better heart.

– Marilyn Vos Savant

Reconstruction is a remarkable, sophisticated procedure. But even the best surgeons in the world can't replace what mastectomy takes away—your own healthy breasts. This chapter explains the cause-and-effect relationship between mastectomy and reconstruction. As you learn how mastectomy is performed, you'll understand what reconstruction can and cannot restore.

The Mastectomy Procedure

Before your operation, your surgeon will use a marking pen to draw the incision lines on your breast. He may do this in the office the day before your surgery, or just before you go into the operating room. He'll also mark around any recent biopsy scar, which will be *re-excised* during surgery. This means cutting around and removing the scar, just in case any cancerous cells remain.

Mastectomy surgery. The following text explains how each step of the mastectomy procedure affects the reconstructed breast.

1. Once you're asleep on the operating table, the surgeon makes incisions along the markings.

Effect: Incisions leave permanent scars. Some may be less conspicuous than others and most fade in time, but scars never disappear completely.

2. The surgeon removes the skin within the incision, including your nipple and areola. This is standard procedure, because most breast cells begin in the ducts, and the ducts converge in the nipple. When patients have non-invasive tumors, or when they have prophylactic mastectomies, some surgeons leave the nipple in place or reuse it after scraping it clean of tissue. Most experts, however, believe this *nipple-sparing* technique leaves potentially harmful cells behind.

Effect: Reconstructed nipples lack the nerve endings or muscle fibers to receive sensation. Therefore, they don't respond to touch or cold the way natural nipples do. Chapter 14 describes nipple reconstruction.

3. The surgeon separates the breast tissue from the skin and underlying muscle and removes as much as possible. This area of tissue extends from under the collarbone to the bottom of the rib cage, and from the breastbone in the middle of the chest to the underarm. Because breast tissue blends with other tissue in the chest, it's not possible to remove it all. That's why a small risk—less than two percent—of breast cancer remains after mastectomy.

Effect: Because nerves are severed when tissue is removed, much of the area remains permanently numb, whether the breast is reconstructed or not. Some nerves do regenerate. The younger you are when you have a mastectomy, the more sensation you're likely to regain. Many women recover some feeling in the upper portion or outer perimeter of the breast, but it is minimal at best. The front of the breast typically remains numb. Women with tissue flaps often regain more sensation in their reconstructed breasts than those with implants.

Effect: Without the cushion of breast tissue, your ribs will be closer to the skin and your underarm may be somewhat indented.

Effect: Removing breast tissue also eliminates ducts and lobules. You can't breastfeed after mastectomy, even if your breast and nipple are reconstructed, because you no longer have the mechanism to produce or deliver milk to the nipple.

Immediate Reconstruction

Women who are in good mental and physical health can have reconstruction, whether it is *immediate* (done as soon as the mastectomy is complete, while you're still asleep on the operating table) or *delayed* (performed as a separate operation anytime after mastectomy). Although 75 percent of women who have reconstruction do so immediately, some are still unaware of their reconstructive choices. One-third of 700 primary care physicians who were surveyed said they didn't refer breast cancer patients to plastic surgeons because they (the physicians) didn't know enough about reconstruction and weren't sure which women were candidates.

> *My oncologist suggested I wait a few months after my mastectomy to see how I felt about reconstruction. But I so feared looking down and seeing nothing but a flat, scarred chest. If I was going to lose my breast, I wanted to replace it as soon as possible. – Diana*

The benefits of immediate reconstruction. For many years, oncologists preferred to delay reconstruction for up to two years after mastectomy to see if the tumor returned. We now know reconstruction does not affect recurrence. While very good results can be achieved when reconstruction is delayed, immediate reconstruction offers distinct benefits:

- Most of your breast skin is preserved.

- Your mastectomy incision is shorter and less obvious.

- You wake up from surgery with a breast mound in place, so you never experience a completely flat chest.

- Combining two procedures—mastectomy and reconstruction—into one operation saves you from going through anesthesia and recovery a second time. It's also less expensive.

If you have immediate reconstruction, your general surgeon and plastic surgeon will coordinate your surgery date. They'll also agree how the mastectomy incision will be made to best accommodate your reconstruction. The general surgeon performs your mastectomy, and while you're still under anesthesia, the plastic surgeon does the reconstruction. Some breast surgeons are qualified to perform both operations.

Skin-sparing mastectomy. When reconstruction is done immediately, a *skin-sparing* mastectomy is often performed. The areola and nipple are removed, but most of the remaining breast skin is preserved to hold and shape your reconstructed breast. Removing the nipple leaves a hole in the breast, through which the entire mastectomy and reconstruction are performed. If you're having an implant procedure, the hole will be filled with a small skin graft from another part of your body.

If your breast will be reconstructed with your own tissue, a portion of the flap will fill the hole. A skin-sparing mastectomy is appropriate unless a patient has tumors in multiple areas of the breast or in the skin itself.

A skin-sparing mastectomy combined with immediate reconstruction often produces a new breast with almost no visible scars. When the new areola is in place, the tiny incision scars are almost complete hidden. A woman going into mastectomy and reconstruction without scarred breasts emerges much the same way. An additional incision to the side or below the nipple is often needed to reach the lymph nodes, remove a large tumor, or when the breast is large or sags a great deal.

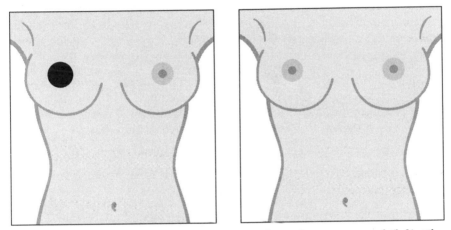

In a skin-sparing mastectomy, the nipple and areola are removed (left). The reconstructed breast often appears unscarred (right).

Delayed Reconstruction

While immediate reconstruction has many advantages, your breast can be rebuilt with good results a month, a year, or 20 years after your mastectomy. Even women who had radical mastectomies when reconstruction wasn't an option can now have new breasts.

If you're not going to have immediate reconstruction, a skin-sparing procedure isn't practical—you'd be left with a lot of baggy skin on your chest. When reconstruction is delayed, the same amount of breast tissue is removed, but a longer horizontal or slanting mastectomy incision is made from below the armpit across the breast. The nipple, areola, and most of the breast skin are removed. The remaining skin is pulled together and stitched closed.

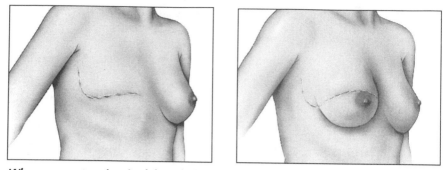

When reconstruction is delayed, the mastectomy scar spans the chest (left). It remains after reconstruction (right), but fades in time.

A mastectomy scar is permanent. If you decide to reconstruct in the future, the surgeon will open your mastectomy scar to accommodate an expander or tissue flap. The scar can't be completely removed from your reconstructed breast, but it will fade considerably in time.

Dealing with chemotherapy and mastectomy was overwhelming. I just couldn't deal with reconstruction issues and decisions. But I changed my mind three years later when I still couldn't face myself in the mirror and I was uncomfortable being naked around my husband. Delaying reconstruction was the right decision for me.
– Copper

When it's best to delay reconstruction. While most women prefer immediate reconstruction, sometimes it's not practical or prudent. It's best to delay when you:

- Have an existing health condition that may add to your surgical risk or impede healing.

- Are too overwhelmed with your cancer and mastectomy to deal with reconstruction issues and decisions.

- Are still unsure about reconstruction at the time of your mastectomy, or you want to try a prosthesis first.

- Are advised by your doctor to complete chemotherapy, radiation, or other cancer treatments before reconstruction.

Coordinating Reconstruction with Adjuvant Therapies

While reconstruction can be of tremendous psychological benefit, treating your cancer is always your medical team's first priority. They may recommend mastectomy in combination with chemotherapy, radiation, or other treatments: *neoadjuvant* (before mastectomy) treatment generally doesn't affect the timing of reconstruction.

Adjuvant (after mastectomy) treatment may limit your options for immediate reconstruction.

In almost all cases involving adjuvant therapy, an expander or implant can be placed at the time of mastectomy. Flap reconstruction may be delayed, particularly if you need to begin chemotherapy or radiation as soon as possible—you don't want to postpone treatment if you're slow to heal or develop complications. The timing of each woman's reconstruction is evaluated individually. Discuss your own reconstruction with your oncologist, radiologist, surgeon, and other physicians involved in your treatment.

Chemotherapy. In some cases, adjuvant chemotherapy can be delayed for six weeks while the implant expansion process is completed. If your doctor prefers to begin chemotherapy right away, the expander can be inflated during your treatment. If you don't feel up to it, you can delay expansion until you complete your chemo regimen. Exchanging the expander for an impant and creating a new nipple must wait until your immune system recovers—usually three to six months after your final session. Flap reconstruction might be delayed until chemotherapy is completed.

I was disappointed when my oncologist said I should delay reconstruction for at least a year after my mastectomy. Intellectually, I knew chemo was more important, but emotionally, I didn't want to be without breasts. I'm glad I waited, because it gave me time to think about my options. – Sarah

Radiation. The best reconstruction involves skin that hasn't been radiated, but we don't always have that luxury. Adjuvant radiation is sometimes appropriate to destroy residual cancer cells after mastectomy. Although it is effective, radiation reduces elasticity and circulation in the skin. Implant and expander reconstruction produce better results and fewer complications when performed before the skin is irradiated. In most cases, the expansion process can be completed quickly, and the expander can be exchanged for an implant prior to adjuvant radiation.

Flap reconstruction produces better results when performed *after* radiation. Several research projects have confirmed this, including a significant 10-year study by the M.D. Anderson Cancer Clinic. It found patients who had immediate flap reconstruction followed by radiation had an 87.5 percent complication rate compared to 8.6 percent for those who had radiation before flap reconstruction.

Other adjuvant therapies. Other treatments that may be prescribed don't usually affect or interfere with reconstruction. Hormone therapies reduce or eliminate the estrogen some breast cancer cells need to survive. Tamoxifen is an anti-estrogen therapy commonly precscribed to reduce the risk of new cancers and recurrence in both pre-menopausal and post-menopausal women. Faslodex treats post-menopausal women who have metastatic cancer. Raloxifene, an anti-osteoporosis drug, shows promise for reducing breast cancer risk. Arimidex, Femara, Aromasin, and other hormone therapy drugs are *aromatase inhibitors.* They benefit post-menopausal women with breast cancer by stopping the body from converting other hormones to estrogen (which it does after menopause). Immune therapy prompts a patient's own system to destroy cancer cells.

Chapter 5

Considering Prophylactic Mastectomy

Whenever you look for a helping hand,
look first at the end of your arm.

– Unknown

Ironically, we've come full circle with regard to mastectomy. In an era of early detection and breast conservation, more women are now choosing to remove their healthy breasts. Prophylactic mastectomy is the most drastic action a woman can take to reduce her risk of breast cancer. It's also the most effective. And it's controversial. While experts agree removing most breast tissue removes most risk, some are concerned too many women needlessly remove their breasts and never would have developed breast cancer anyway.

Why would a woman choose to remove her perfectly healthy breasts? Because she's convinced they are ticking time bombs and the risk they will go off is simply too scary to live with. Perhaps she's lost her mother to cancer and wants to spare her own child that experience. Maybe she's seen her mother, sister, aunt—or all three—struggle with the disease, and she's prepared to take any possible action to improve her own odds. Women who face unilateral mastectomy may wonder about their opposite breast. Will it too develop cancer sometime in the future? Should they remove it now and be done with it?

No one knows who will get breast cancer and who won't. No one can tell you whether you should remove your healthy breast or not. Only you know what will give you peace of mind. Clearly understanding your risk for developing the disease can help you make the decision.

What would you say your risk is of developing breast cancer? 10 percent? 50 percent? The fact is, most women greatly overstate their risk. Many feel it's only a matter of time before they hear, "You have breast cancer." While fear is a powerful motivator, experience is even stronger. Overstated risk is a hard sell to women who have seen friends or relatives struggle with the disease. For them, the risk can be unbearable.

The results of one study at Sunnybrook and Women's College Health Sciences Centre in Toronto underscore this common overstatement of risk. Sixty women who were about to have prophylactic bilateral mastectomies were asked to estimate their breast cancer risk:

Average risk estimated by participants:	76%
Actual lifetime risk of participants: (women with inherited genetic mutations*)	59%
Actual lifetime risk of participants: (women without inherited genetic mutations*)	17%

Refers to increased hereditary risk discussed later in this chapter.

Would you change your mind about prophylactic mastectomy if you knew your estimated risk was 17 percent? Put another way: your chance of NOT getting breast cancer would be 83 percent.

Making Sense of Statistics

To say breast cancer risk is a complex subject is a gross understatement. While researchers continue to make great strides in understanding the disease, there is still much to discover. Until we know what causes it, we can't predict who will get it or who won't. The best we can do to estimate an individual's risk is to determine the rate at which the disease occurs in women of similar age, then increase or decrease that statistic by an individual's own family history, genetics, and lifestyle factors.

The dreaded one-in-eight. The "one-in-eight" statistic we often hear is probably the most misunderstood. It represents the *absolute risk* of developing breast cancer for women over age 80. That means one of eight women who live beyond that age will be diagnosed with breast cancer during her lifetime.

Absolute risk is determined by counting the number of women of similar age who develop breast cancer. The number is meaningless unless it's applied to a specific timeframe—one, five, or 20 years, for example. The following table shows a woman has a one-in-54 chance of developing breast cancer by the time she's 50. Conversely, the likelihood she'll remain free of the disease by that age is greater than 98 percent. Her risk increases as she ages.

Absolute Risk for Developing Breast Cancer		
AGE		LIFETIME RISK
by age 30	one in 2,212	(<1.0%)
by age 40	one in 235	(<1.0%)
by age 50	one in 54	(1.85%)
by age 60	one in 23	(4.34%)
by age 70	one in 14	(7.14%)
by age 80	one in 10	(10.0%)
beyond age 80	one in 8	(12.5%)

Source: National Cancer Institute

Risk Factors

A risk factor is something that increases your chance of developing a disease. Having additional risk factors for breast cancer doesn't guarantee you'll develop disease; it means you're more likely to do so. Most women who are diagnosed have no known risk factors. Many women with several risk factors never develop the disease.

Consider a hypothetical illustration of how your own risk factors might influence your absolute risk. If one of every eight American women weighs 150 pounds by age 50, does that mean you will? Not necessarily. The risk for individuals is different, because their personal risk factors are not the same. Factors you can control (diet and exercise)

> *I could never bring myself to remove a perfectly healthy breast. I'm very diligent in doing self-exams and mammograms. I'm confident we would catch anything early enough to treat. Besides, there might be a cure by then.*
> – Faith

and those you can't (genetics) play an important role in determining your weight at any given age.

The same rationale applies to your chance of getting breast cancer. Your own risk factors increase or decrease the absolute risk for your age group—something to keep in mind the next time the nightly news teases with "a woman is diagnosed with breast cancer every two minutes."

Risk factors you can't control. Each of the following risk factors is thought to increase your chance of developing breast cancer. Researchers suspect other risk factors are yet to be discovered.

- Gender. Although 1,500 men develop breast cancer each year, every woman is at risk simply by virtue of her sex.

- Race. Breast cancer occurs predominantly in non-Hispanic Caucasian women. Women of African-American descent are less likely to develop it, but if they do, are more likely to die from it. Hispanic and Asian women have lower rates of the disease.

- Age. Our risk increases as we grow older. This may partially explain the rise in breast cancer rates over the past few years: 77 percent of all breast cancers occur in women age 50 and older, and our population is aging.

- Family history. If a first-degree blood relative (mother, sister, or daughter) had breast cancer before age 50, your risk is two to three times higher than someone without the same family history. It's important to put this in context: if the absolute lifetime risk is two percent for a woman of your age without a family history of breast cancer, your lifetime risk is four to six percent. If more than one first-degree relative had breast cancer, your risk is four to five times greater.

- Inherited gene mutations. There's a difference between *genetic* and *hereditary*. All cancers are genetic, meaning they originate in the genes. Hereditary breast cancers usually occur before age 50 and are caused by gene mutations passed along from one or both parents. If you've inherited a particular gene mutation (see "Genetic Testing" later in this chapter), your lifetime risk of developing breast cancer may be 50 to 85 percent higher than someone without the same mutation. Less than 10 percent of breast cancers are hereditary.

- Previous breast cancer. If you have previously had breast cancer, your risk of developing it again is about one percent per year— that's 20 percent over the next 20 years. Younger women have a higher risk, as do those with a family history of breast cancer.

- Prior radiation. Your risk is increased if your chest was irradiated for any reason before age 20.

- Estrogen exposure. Many breast cancers thrive on estrogen. The longer your body is exposed to the hormone, the greater your risk. Menstruation before age 12 or menopause after age 50 increases your risk by two or three times above average. Taking hormone replacement therapy may also increase risk (see "Hormone replacement therapy" below).

- Environmental factors. Carcinogens in our water, food, and environment may cause normal cells to mutate and become cancerous. This may partially explain why people in urban locations are more likely to develop breast cancer than those in more undeveloped areas. Breast cancer rates are significantly higher, for example, in New York and California than in Alaska and Wyoming.

Risk factors you can control. Now, the good news. You can control several lifestyle factors thought to increase your risk of breast cancer, including the following.

- Pregnancy. Women who never have children, never breastfeed, or have children after age 30 are at higher risk due to prolonged estrogen exposure.

- Hormone replacement therapy (HRT). Although women have taken HRT for decades to minimize the effects of menopause and protect against heart disease, the Women's Health Initiative was the first comprehensive clinical study to assess the related risks and benefits. The study was halted prematurely in 2002 when daily doses of combined estrogen and progestin were found to increase breast cancer risk slightly. Participants' risk returned to normal six months after they stopped taking HRT.

- Birth control pills. Most studies show no significant increased risk from taking birth control pills, regardless of the estrogen dosage or length of use. Surprised? Birth control pills were thought to be a major culprit when estrogen was found to stimulate some breast cancers. However, most studies show oral contraceptives increase risk to a very small degree, if at all. These minimally elevated risk levels return to normal 10 years after women stop taking the Pill.

- Lifestyle factors. More and more studies are linking exercise and weight control with reduced risk for breast cancer and many other diseases. Overweight women are at higher risk, especially after menopause, when their fat tissue can convert some hormones into estrogen. Although researchers suspect certain foods increase the probability of breast cancer, no conclusive evidence shows whether a particular diet promotes the disease or protects against it. The jury is still out on soy. Despite its popularity, we don't know if plant estrogen increases or reduces breast cancer risk. Until more definitive evidence is available, experts recommend following a sensible, balanced diet with plenty of lean protein, fiber, fresh fruit, and vegetables. Because alcohol inhibits the liver's ability to regulate estrogen in the blood, it's a known risk factor; the question is to what degree. Drinking less than five servings of alcohol per week probably doesn't increase risk significantly.

Genetic Testing

If the one-in-eight statistic is the most misunderstood aspect of breast cancer, genetic testing is a close second. Lately, this testing is getting a lot of attention. Unfortunately, a 1,000-word article or a 60-second news story isn't usually enough to tell the whole story. This misinformation fuels speculation of women prophylactically removing their breasts because of overstated risk. ("Are too many women removing their breasts needlessly? News at 11.")

I lost my grandmother to breast cancer, and my mother died of the disease when I was 12. That's all the data I need. If losing my breasts means my daughter will be spared that horrible experience, then so be it. – Monica

Genetics is an incredibly important, if relatively new and complex field. We know it's the key to understanding breast cancer: we just don't know how or why. In 1990, researchers made a giant leap forward when they discovered the BReast CAncer 1 (BRCA1) gene. In 1994, they discovered BReast CAncer 2 (BRCA2), a less common gene. When these BRCA genes are healthy, they produce proteins to repair cell damage and prevent potentially cancerous cells from forming. When a woman's BRCA genes mutate and no longer function in this protective role, she is at increased risk for developing breast and ovarian cancers.

Although we often hear so-and-so is being tested to see if she has the "breast cancer" gene, this is a misnomer, since we all have BRCA1/2. Genetic testing attempts to determine whether you have a mutation of these genes.

All men and women have two copies of BRCA1 and two copies of BRCA2. We inherit one copy from each parent. Either side can pass along a mutation. If your mother or father had a BRCA1 and BRCA2 mutation, there's a 50 percent chance it was passed to you. Likewise, if you have one or both of these mutations, you have a 50 percent chance of passing it on to your daughter. BRCA gene mutations increase the risk for developing:

- A first case of breast cancer by age 70.

- Breast cancer in the opposite breast (if already diagnosed in one breast).

- Ovarian cancer.

Implications of test results. Why wouldn't every woman want to rush out and get tested? Because it's expensive—as much as $2,800, depending on the type of testing—and often not covered by health insurance.

Chemotherapy and radiation for my left breast convinced me I never wanted to repeat the experience. Finding I had the BRCA1 mutation reinforced my decision to have the right side removed. I don't regret what I did, and I don't worry every time a new study comes out. I made my decision on the best data available at the time. – Dana

The testing can't predict whether you will or won't get breast cancer, but it can provide data that may help you decide whether to keep or remove your healthy breast. But not everyone needs to be tested. Since 90 percent or more of breast cancers are *not* hereditary, most women will test negative for BRCA1 and BRCA2. Testing is appropriate for women with a personal or family history of breast or ovarian cancer, those of Ashkenazi Jewish descent, or women with certain other high risk factors.

While scientists know where to look for most of the BRCA1/2 markers in the blood, others are unknown. That means if you do test negative (as most women will), you may still have the abnormality, but current testing limitations can't identify it, and you may still develop breast cancer. You may have other as-yet unidentified mutations. If you have a BRCA mutation, you're at greater risk, but a positive test doesn't guarantee you'll develop the disease.

Researchers are still looking for other genes that may increase breast cancer risk. Recent discovery of the CHEK2 gene, for example, may help discover what causes breast cancer in women who have a family history of the disease but don't have BRCA1 or BRCA2. In 2003, scientists discovered the BP1 gene, which may be present in 80 percent of breast cancer tumors. Hopefully, this discovery will lead to

My genetic testing confirmed my worst fears: I'm positive for BRCA1 and BRCA2. In a weird way, I feel somewhat relieved knowing, rather than suspecting, I had the mutations. – Avita

improved methods of early detection and treatment. As we learn more about genetic influences on breast cancer, we'll be better able to predict individual risk.

Genetic Counseling

Although any physician can order genetic testing, it takes a qualified expert to interpret the results and estimate an individual's overall risk for breast cancer. Genetic counselors (also called medical geneticists) have specialized graduate degrees. They can explain the benefits and limitations of genetic testing and determine if testing is appropriate for you. If your oncologist, surgeon, or other physician recommends genetic testing, ask for a referral to a genetic counselor.

Genetic counseling begins with your complete medical and family history. You can prepare for your session by documenting any cancers, and the age at which they occurred, within three or four generations on both sides of the family.

To find a genetic counselor, ask your oncologist or plastic surgeon for a referral, contact the National Society of Genetic Counselors (610-872-7608 or www.nsgc.org), or the National Cancer Institute (800-4-cancer or www.cancer.gov). For more information on the benefits and risks of genetic testing, see the National Cancer Institute's website. Another excellent resource is *Assess Your True Risk of Breast Cancer* by Patricia T. Kelly, Ph.D. (www.ptkelly.com).

If you decide to be tested, a sample of your blood will be sent to Myriad Genetics (800-725-2722 or www.myriad.com), the only testing source in the United States. In about three weeks, your genetic counselor will receive the test results and explain what they mean. She can't tell you whether you will or won't develop breast cancer, but she can better estimate your risk.

Paying for genetic counseling and testing. While many health insurers won't pay for genetic counseling or testing, some will if the ordering physician requests it and identifies you as high risk. Myriad offers a no-charge pre-authorization service to determine whether your insurance will pay for the cost of your test. You should know that many insurance companies consider prophylactic mastectomy unnecessary, and will not pay for the procedure. There's more on this in Chapter 7.

Although the Health Insurance Portability and Accountability Act prohibits health carriers from denying coverage to anyone with group insurance because of genetic test information, some women prefer to pay for the testing themselves rather than risk discrimination.

Making Your Decision

While no one wants to lose her breasts, some women at high risk may consider prophylactic mastectomy a no-brainer. They want to do everything they can to reduce the likelihood of getting breast cancer. Other women would never consider removing their healthy breasts. For most, the decision is tortuous. Should they? Shouldn't they? Whatever your circumstances, prophylactic mastectomy is a deeply personal act. Even when you know your personal risk factors, it may be difficult to make your decision. If we all wore helmets while we drove, we would reduce our risk of injury on the road, but how many of us are willing to do that?

If you're considering prophylactic mastectomy, try to temper your emotion with information. The following four steps will help lead you to decision you can live with:

Determine your overall risk. There's a world of difference between fear and high-risk. The threat of breast cancer is frightening, but prophylactic surgery is a big decision. Once done, it can't be undone. Before you act, understand your estimated annual and lifetime risks.

Consider your tolerance for risk. Remember, it's your combined risk for developing breast cancer over your lifetime that's most important. While one woman might consider a 35 percent risk intolerable, another may find it acceptable. Try this exercise if you decide to have genetic counseling: write down your least tolerable risk percentage. This would be your deal-breaker—the lowest risk at which you would seriously consider prophylactic mastectomy. Then compare that number to the estimated risk provided by your geneticist. This may help to reinforce your decision or change your mind about losing your breast.

Consider the alternatives. If you're at increased risk for breast cancer, prophylactic mastectomy is not your only option. You may want to consider close monitoring: annual mammograms, biannual professional examinations, and monthly self-breast exams—to detect any future breast cancer at an early, treatable stage. Additional monitoring may include magnetic resonance imaging (MRI) or *ductal lavage,* a new, non-surgical Pap smear of the nipple for high-risk women (this procedure is described in Chapter 21). Tamoxifen may also be an appropriate preventative treatment. Another option is to participate in a clinical trial for high-risk women (visit www.nci.nih.gov).

If you test positive for a BRCA mutation and aren't planning to have children, you may want to consider *oophorectomy*—prophylactic removal of your ovaries—to greatly reduce the amount of estrogen in your body. Oophorectomy reduces the risk of ovarian cancer by 95 percent and risk of breast cancer by 50 percent in women with BRCA mutations. If you're still having menstrual periods, oophorectomy will force your body into menopause.

Make a decision you won't regret. Ultimately, whether you do or don't proceed with prophylactic mastectomy is your decision. Everyone you know—family, friends, and medical professionals—will have their own opinions about what you should do. The wisest course of action is to gather all the information you need to make a decision that's right for you.

Finding Answers, Making Decisions

Chapter 6

Finding Dr. Right

*If you can't hug your doctor,
you've got the wrong one.*

– Kay, breast cancer patient

As a breast cancer patient, you have a small army of medical professionals supporting and treating you. But when it comes to reconstruction, your surgeon takes center stage.

Any competent surgeon can remove a breast. Rebuilding one is not as easy. It takes skill and experience to tailor reconstruction to each woman's unique needs. A good surgeon is an artist and a sculptor—a post-mastectomy chest is his canvas and clay. Your new breasts are quite literally in his hands. He does the work, but you live with it.

Reconstruction may be one of the most personal decisions you'll ever make. If you're going to go through the effort, it makes sense to find a surgeon with whom you feel confident and comfortable. This does take a bit more effort on your part. Just when you're the most vulnerable, you must make decisions about reconstruction—decisions that may affect you for the rest of your life. Some women are relieved to let the surgeon worry about how their reconstruction will be performed. They consult with one surgeon, perhaps chosen from the telephone directory, and agree to whatever he recommends. That's an easy decision, but one a woman may later regret.

Caveat Emptor

"Buyer beware" is good advice when considering the services of any professional, including surgeons. The first surgeon you see may give you a great result. Then again, he might not. You probably wouldn't choose the first lawyer, financial advisor, realtor, or other professional you found. It's the same with surgeons. They're human like the rest of us; and being human, they have different personalities, skills, and opinions about how reconstruction can be accomplished. Some are great at their craft but lousy with people. You may feel utterly uncomfortable with one, while another fills you with confidence. You're most likely to be satisfied with your new breast when you consider more than one surgeon and evaluate different reconstructive techniques.

> *The mastectomy surgeon recommended a plastic surgeon, and that's who I saw. He told me how he would rebuild my breasts and I agreed. Months later, I spoke to another woman who had reconstruction with an entirely different technique that sounded much better. Why didn't my surgeon mention that one? – Lanie*

When a surgeon downplays one technique or the other, it may be because he feels it's not in your best interest, or because he isn't experienced doing it. For example, if the first surgeon you see only does implant reconstruction, he may not mention the possibility of a tissue flap. A surgeon qualified to do the TRAM flap, a tissue transfer that uses abdominal fat and muscle, may not explain the DIEP procedure, an improved technique that preserves the muscle and has fewer side effects. (TRAM and DIEP procedures are described in Chapter 11.)

Four Characteristics of an Ideal Plastic Surgeon

When you consider different surgeons, look for four important characteristics:

Skill. There's no such thing as a typical reconstruction, because each woman is different. It takes skill and experience to rebuild and fine-tune a breast to get the shape and symmetry right. Never judge a surgeon's skill by his brochure or website. Depend on his qualifications, feedback from other patients, photos of his work, and your own confidence in him.

Compassion. You're more than a statistic on a chart, and you deserve to be treated as an individual. A good surgeon cares about your expectations. He is sympathetic to your concerns and reacts to your anxiety with compassion.

Rapport. It's important to find a surgeon with a personality to match your own. One surgeon may be too aggressive, another too impersonal for your taste. Your surgeon should talk with you, not to you, and give you his undivided attention. He ought to care what you want and answer your questions patiently, even when you ask him to repeat something.

Honesty. Look for a surgeon who describes what you can realistically expect, rather than what he thinks you want to hear. If you have your heart set on D-cup implants, he should tell you whether your skin can be expanded sufficiently to accommodate that size. If you're leaning toward a tissue flap, he ought to describe what you can expect from the operation, recovery, and how you'll look afterward. Think twice if a surgeon promises, "You'll be good as new," or "Your breasts will be perfect."

My surgeon put me at ease by patiently answering all my questions. He smiled a lot, spoke slowly, and explained several different ways the reconstruction might be done. I felt I was talking to a trusted friend. – Cameran

I was so put off by my surgeon, I skipped my last appointment. He was more interested in me as his "creation" than as a person with cancer. He refused to accept that I didn't want big breasts! – Alicia

Shopping for a Surgeon

The best way to find a great surgeon is to solicit referrals, then conduct your own interviews with at least two or three before deciding on one. Be selective. Personal feedback is always preferable to the "eeney-meeney-miney-moe" method.

The general surgeon who does your mastectomy will probably refer you to a local reconstructive surgeon. Ask your oncologist, gynecologist, and other medical professionals for recommendations. Breast cancer nurses are also great sources of information. Hospitals and teaching universities often have departments devoted specifically to breast cancer surgery, and many have excellent reconstruction staff.

The best referrals come from satisfied customers. It's always nice to hear an endorsement from someone who's been through reconstruction, preferably the same technique you're considering. Ask other women who they do or don't recommend and why. Reach to Recovery (800-227-2345) will put you in touch with women in your area who will share their insights into the reconstruction experience and give you feedback about their plastic surgeons. Choose a surgeon who specializes in breast reconstruction. You don't want your new breast made by a hand surgeon who reconstructs only one or two breasts a year.

Will you settle for good if you can get great? The best reconstructive opportunity isn't always available locally, particularly if you live in a small town or rural area. The closest surgeon may be on the other side of the city or in the next state. Maybe you want a flap reconstruction, but the local surgeons only do implant procedures. If the surgeons and techniques you want aren't available nearby, will you travel to get what you want or will you settle for the local expertise?

If you want nothing but the best, you may need to pack up and spend a few days or several weeks at a renowned facility, such as M.D. Anderson in Houston, U.C.L.A. in Los Angeles, or Memorial Sloan Kettering Cancer Center in New York, to get one of the best surgeons or the most advanced technique. The DIEP tissue transfer mentioned earlier is a good example. Few U.S. doctors are qualified to perform this technically advanced procedure. Many women who want the best possible flap reconstruction consider the cost and effort involved in traveling to one of these experts well worth the result.

Insurance restrictions. Managed care organizations may insist you choose a surgeon within their network of providers. Other policies may pay all or a portion of the cost, no matter whom you choose. If you can show the procedure you want is not available locally, the insurer may negotiate with the surgeon to cover your operation. Some plastic surgeons are willing to do this, but many others won't, since health insurers typically pay considerably less than surgeons' usual fees. Chapter 7 provides more information about paying for reconstruction.

Before You Schedule an Appointment

Make a list of the surgeons others recommend. Then do a little homework before your appointment, to make the most of your time with the surgeon.

Know what you want. Your plastic surgeon may be a primary source of information, but he shouldn't be your only source. Nor should you depend on him to give you a tutorial on reconstruction. Use this book and the research techniques described in Chapter 7 to learn about reconstructive terms and procedures. Answer as many of your own questions as you can. Weigh the advantages and disadvantages of implants compared to tissue flaps.

Verify certification. The ASPS is the largest professional organization of reconstructive surgeons. To be certified, a surgeon must graduate from an accredited medical school, complete a five-year residency of general and plastic surgery, practice for at least two years, and successfully complete oral and written exams. In most states—here's a frightening thought—*any* licensed physician can legally perform plastic surgery. While certification doesn't guarantee proficiency, it's a good starting place. Call the ASPS or use the "Find a Surgeon" feature on the organization's website (www.plasticsurgery.org or 800-635-0635) for breast reconstruction specialists in your area.

The Consultation

Good plastic surgeons keep busy. If you can't get an appointment with a particular surgeon as soon as you would like, be sure to tell the receptionist how much time you have before your mastectomy. They will often try to fit you in. In the meantime, see other surgeons and continue your research.

Most surgeons begin by reviewing the patient's cancer diagnosis, treatment, and overall medical history. They'll show you their portfolios of before-and-after patient photos. Usually, this will only reflect their best work. Ask to see photos of the not-so-good reconstructions as well, to get a broader perspective of possible reconstructive results. The surgeon will check the quality and amount of your breast skin, and if you're considering a tissue flap, he'll determine whether you have sufficient tissue at the donor site. Here are a few tips for making the most of your appointment.

Bring your medical records. When you schedule an appointment, ask whether you should bring your pathology reports, mammograms, or other medical records for review. Then contact your doctor's office, hospital, or other facility to gather up everything you need. You'll need to return the items after your consultation appointments.

Disclose all the medications, vitamins, and herbs you take. Your surgeon will advise which, if any, you should discontinue before surgery and when you can resume taking them (generally a couple of weeks after surgery). This is very important, because some may interfere with circulation or healing. Include all prescribed and over-the-counter items. If you have several items to disclose, it's easier to hand your surgeon a list like the following:

Sample List of Medications			
MEDICATION	STRENGTH	FREQUENCY	REASON
Celebrex	100 mg	twice daily	arthritis
Premarin	.625 mg	once daily	HRT
Aspirin	.325 mg	1-2 times weekly	headache, back pain
Black cohosh	370 mg		menopause
Multivitamin		once daily	general health

Arrange for someone to come with you. There will be lots of information to absorb, and four ears are better than two.

Don't be afraid to communicate. The most successful consultation is interactive. Describe what you want from reconstruction and voice your concerns. If you want your breasts to look as they do before mastectomy, tell the surgeon. If you would like smaller, larger, or rounder breasts, now is the time to say so. Don't be afraid to speak up if you need something explained, spelled or repeated. Ask your surgeon to draw you a picture to clarify a procedure. Inquire about anything that concerns or confuses you, no matter how silly or insignificant it may seem. He's probably heard it all before, but he knows it's all new to you.

> *My mother's generation didn't question authority, so she never asked her doctor what to expect from her mastectomy—and he didn't tell her. The poor woman was filled with fear, when a couple of simple questions would have saved her from the horrors of her own imagination. – Eberly*

Take notes. You'll have lots of questions for your surgeon, and it's easy to be overwhelmed by new information, especially if you're nervous or uncomfortable. Write down the key points of your discussion so you can review them later. If someone accompanies you, he or she can take notes while you focus on listening. Or tape your discussion for later review.

Let it all sink in. Never feel pressured to make a decision about a surgeon or operation while in the office. Take time to think about what you've heard. Let everything sink in. Discuss your options with someone you trust to get another perspective. After your appointment, follow up to learn more about new terms or techniques you may have heard. Ask to be put in touch with one or two patients who had the same procedure you're considering.

The following questions will help you assess and compare the different ways surgeons approach reconstruction. If surgeons don't discuss these issues during your consultation appointments, be sure to ask.

Questions for Your Plastic Surgeon

- Which reconstruction option is best for me and why?
- How many reconstructive surgeries of this type have you performed?
- How many surgeries and office visits will be required over what period of time?
- How do you reconstruct the areola and nipple?
- How many scars will I have, and where will they be?
- What's the best result I can expect?
- How long will the surgery, hospital stay, and recovery be?
- When will I be able to return to work?
- What will my recovery be like?
- What are the side effects and risks?
- How will you make sure my reconstructed breast and natural breast are symmetrical?
- What if I'm not satisfied with the results?
- How much will this cost? (if you're paying for any of the cost)

The Value of a Second (or Third) Opinion

My surgeon gave me his full attention, spending more than an hour answering all my questions. I felt as though I were his only patient. When he was late during my subsequent appointments, I remained unperturbed, imagining him patiently dealing with another woman in my situation. – Marilyn

Reconstruction recommendations may vary widely, depending on the experience and skill of the plastic surgeon. You have nothing to lose and everything to gain by getting a second, if not a third, opinion. You won't offend a surgeon; getting another opinion is standard practice when any surgery is involved. You may end up choosing the first surgeon you speak with, but it's good to consider other ideas. Some women see several surgeons before choosing one. At some point, however, you'll have heard all the answers.

If you're uncomfortable with a surgeon for any reason, find someone else. Would you let a realtor talk you into buying a house you disliked? Think the grocer could persuade you to buy a bag of melons you didn't want? Remember, you're doing the hiring. You needn't feel compelled or coerced to have one or the other do your surgery. Keep looking until you're satisfied you've found your surgical partner.

Who pays for other opinions? Most health carriers pay for a second surgeon's opinion. Contact your own insurance company to see if they will cover additional consultation appointments or require pre-authorization from your primary physician.

He or she? Some women feel female surgeons are more sympathetic and can relate to reconstruction issues better than men. Thousands of women who are happy with their male plastic surgeons might disagree. While many breast cancer patients may feel more comfortable with a woman surgeon, it's best to evaluate each surgeon on his or her own merits—you be the judge of what's best for you.

I saw three different surgeons, who recommended three different techniques! One wanted to reconstruct my breast with implants, another wanted to use tissue from my back, and the third said I would have better results using my abdominal fat. – Sondra

Chapter 7

Searching for Answers

You have brains in your head.
You have feet in your shoes.
You can steer yourself
any direction you choose.

– from *Oh, the Places You'll Go!* by Dr. Seuss

You may have a team of medical professionals supporting your breast cancer treatment, but guess who most influences your reconstruction?

You do.

Making your own decisions about reconstruction can restore the lack of control you may feel during your diagnosis and treatment. But you can't make informed decisions without information. So how do you find answers when you're not even sure of the right questions?

Why Bother with Research?

When it comes to surgery, informed is always better than impetuous. Exploring your options gives you the information you need to make the right choices about your reconstruction. You would probably compare loan rates before buying a home or a car, and get to know someone pretty well before you marrying them or forming a business partnership. It's only logical to approach a decision concerning your physical and emotional well-being with the same scrutiny. To use a corny football analogy, don't sit on the bench. Suit up and get in the game. Be your own advocate.

Read the menu before you order. When you dine in a new restaurant, do you read the menu first or take whatever the waiter recommends?

If you don't like your dinner, you can send it back and order something else. Reconstruction offers the same opportunity for personal preference. It will be much more difficult, however, if you don't like your new breast.

Becoming informed gives you the power of choice. Along the way, you may discover reconstruction can give you a better breast than you thought, or that it requires more than you're willing to go through.

The benefits of research. Carefully contemplating all your options provides distinct advantages:

- You eliminate fear of the unknown. Reconstruction can be an exciting *and* terrifying possibility. You can wake up from your mastectomy without ever experiencing a flat chest, but how will you look? How will you feel? What if you aren't satisfied with your results? What are the long-term effects? Your own research will demystify reconstruction, replacing the unknown with the expected. The more you learn about reconstruction, the less anxiety you'll have about the process.

- You make a choice that's right for you. Whether you have reconstruction or not is your decision. No one else can make it for you—not your spouse, partner, doctor, family, or friends with their own reconstruction experiences. You're the one who must go through the surgery and recovery, and you're the one who'll live with the results. You're the one who must make the Big Decision.

- You set realistic expectations. You can never anticipate every possible feeling and experience associated with reconstruction. Once you understand all the advantages and disadvantages of the various reconstructive procedures, however, you're less likely to have unpleasant surprises, because you'll know what to expect.

Eight Tips to Make the Most of Your Research

Investigating reconstruction means more doctor appointments and learning new terms and procedures. Given everything else you've been through with your breast cancer, it can be overwhelming. The following tips will help you stay on track.

1. **Establish a positive attitude about learning.** Consider your research an empowering action rather than an awful chore. Your investigative efforts will help you make a confident decision.

2. **Take time to learn.** Most breast cancers grow for six to eight years before they're large enough to be detected. Unless your cancer is very aggressive, taking three to four weeks to learn about reconstruction probably won't adversely affect your health. If you want to proceed with immediate reconstruction, ask your oncologist how long you can wait before having your mastectomy. If you decide to delay your reconstruction, you can research at your own pace, without the scheduling limitations of mastectomy.

3. **Be patient and persistent.** Take things one step at a time. Don't let frustration get you down. When you think you can't absorb any more information (but need to), take a break. Go to lunch with a friend, listen to your favorite music, see a movie, or go for a walk.

4. **Deal with data.** As much as possible, base your decisions on medical information rather than media hype, personal anecdote, or urban myth. If someone tells you implants aren't safe, check a variety of resources for yourself. If a friend of a friend had a terrible experience with a tissue transfer, it doesn't mean you will.

5. **Enlist a study buddy.** Having someone help with your research saves time and provides a second perspective. Ideally, your spouse or partner is the best one to share this task. It helps him or her understand what's going on while supporting you. If this isn't practical, ask a friend, relative, or someone who's been through it before to assist you.

6. **Take notes.** New terms and information can be awfully confusing. As you research, jot down terms or issues you don't understand. When questions arise, you can always go back and review your notes to refresh your memory.

7. **Know when to stop.** At some point, you need to assess all the data you've gathered, and make your decision. If you're still unsure, it's probably best to delay your reconstruction.

8. **Take time to absorb.** Once you've done all your research, give yourself time to let everything sink in. Take a while to reflect on what you've learned. Go away for the day or the weekend to consider your alternatives before making your decision.

References and Resources

An amazing amount of information about reconstruction is available, if you know where to look for the bits and pieces. Here's a sampling of the resources available to you.

Plastic surgeons. As you learned in the previous chapter, plastic surgeons are primary sources of information on reconstruction, although your time with them is limited. Their before-and-after color photos will illustrate their best reconstructive results.

Show-and-tell books. Each and every woman who contemplates reconstruction wants to know how her new breasts will look. Ten years ago, the only visual resources were grainy black-and-whites in old text books. Now there are excellent color photo collections in which breast cancer patients graciously share their personal experiences with surgery and reconstruction. The following books are available at Amazon.com unless otherwise noted.

The First Look by Amelia Davis and Dr. Nancy Snyderman.

Reconstructing Aphrodite by Terry Lorant and Dr. Loren Eskenazi.

Show Me by the Penn State Milton S. Hershey Medical Center (717-531-2042 or www.pennstatewomenshealth.com/showme).

Winged Victory: Altered Images: Transcending Breast Cancer by Art Myers.

The Internet. With a few clicks of your mouse, you can bring information and personal experiences directly to your desktop. And it's free. A dizzying array of data awaits: research reports, plastic surgeons' websites, full-color photos, and personal reconstruction journals. Begin with the websites listed throughout this book. Use Google (www.google.com) or your favorite search engine to find others. Be as specific as possible to pinpoint the type of reconstruction information you're looking for. Searching for "breast reconstruction" for example, lists 29,300 sources, while a search for "breast expanders" finds 33 sites. Bookmark your favorite websites for easy return.

Internet discussion groups, also called message boards, can provide information and encouragement when you're trying to cope with reconstruction and other cancer issues. Members share tips for preparing for surgery and getting through recovery. Many are very knowledgeable about breast cancer and reconstruction, but remember: their strength is peer support, not medical advice.

One of the most informative and supportive online neighborhoods is the Facing Our Risk of Cancer Empowered (FORCE) website (www.facingourrisk.org). While the site's primary focus is hereditary breast cancer risk, discussions cover a variety of breast cancer subjects. Members have been through every breast cancer and reconstruction experience imaginable. No matter where you are in the reconstruction process, others are ready and willing to share their own experiences and lend a virtual shoulder.

Other online message boards are devoted primarily to breast cancer, but sometimes discuss reconstruction. Try Susan G. Komen Breast Cancer Foundation (www.komen.org), Cancer Support Network (www.acscsn.org) and ivillage (www.ivillagehealth.com/boards).

Tips for Using Online Discussion Groups

- Some groups are more active than others. Notice how frequently messages are posted.

- If a message board has a search feature, use it to find discussions containing the specific words or phrases in which you're most interested, such as "nipple reconstruction."

- Read through the archives of previous postings before submitting questions. It's great research, and chances are someone else has already provided the answers you're looking for.

Individual and group support. What better resource can you have than someone who has been through it all? Doctors can explain clinical details, but women who have been through reconstruction can give you blow-by-blow descriptions and practical information. Given the chance, they're usually more than happy to show-and-tell—they'll share their experiences and may even show you their rebuilt breasts. Ask your plastic surgeon to refer you to one or two previous patients whose circumstances are as close as possible to your own, considering your age, cancer treatment, and the type of reconstructive technique you're considering.

One caveat about this information: women are often passionate about their reconstruction, whether they're happy with the results or not. Everyone is different. Someone else's experience won't necessarily be yours, and her choice may not be the best solution for you. Keep the opinion of others in perspective. Consider their input as part of your overall research. Store it all in the mental information hopper, but never substitute personal opinion for medical advice, or use the experience of just one or two women to make your decision.

Support groups can also be quite helpful. Contact your nearest ACS office, local hospital, breast cancer center, or medical association to see if they sponsor reconstruction discussion groups, workshops, or lectures. You might call the supervisor first, to ask if a particular group discusses reconstruction. The National Alliance of Breast

Cancer Organizations (888-80-NABCO or www.nabco.org) also provides information about local and national support groups.

Libraries and bookstores. You'll find shelves full of breast cancer books, but few include more than a cursory chapter or two on reconstruction. New books will undoubtedly be published and made available in the future. The medical libraries of your hospital, college, or university may offer more information. Call or visit to see what they have on file.

Paying for Your Reconstruction

If you've had a smooth relationship with your insurance company during your treatment, you are among the fortunate. Women frequently say dealing with health insurers is almost as nerve-wracking as coping with cancer. Some patients actually pay for services that should be covered simply to avoid the frustration of dealing with insurance hassles and denied claims.

Your rights as a breast cancer patient. In 1998, 84 percent of ASPS member physicians reported having patients who were denied coverage for breast reconstruction. Fortunately, the Women's Health and Cancer Rights Act (WHCRA) took effect the following year. This law requires health companies to pay for the following:

- Breast prostheses.
- Breast reconstruction after mastectomy.
- Surgery to the other breast to achieve a symmetrical appearance.
- Treatment for complications from mastectomy or reconstruction.

Two particular circumstances are exempt from the WHCRA mandate. The law doesn't require insurance companies to pay for mastectomies; but if they do, they must also pay for reconstruction. Coverage is not retroactive. If you weren't insured with your current plan before January 1999 when the WHCRA took effect, or you had your mastectomy before that time, your insurer is not obligated to cover your reconstruction.

To learn more about the WHCRA, contact the Department of Labor, Pensions, and Welfare Benefits Administration (800-998-7542 or www.askebsa.dol.gov). Type in "whcra" in the search box to find the publication. Many states have additional laws regarding mastectomy and reconstruction. Contact your Congressional representative or your state's Department of Health.

What's covered, what's not. If a health plan covers mastectomy and reconstruction, it must do so under its overall guidelines. You still have to pay any deductibles and co-payments routinely required for office visits or other services, but you cannot be required to pay more solely for breast cancer surgeries. In other words, if your Blue Shield coverage normally pays 80 percent of medical services and you pay the remaining 20 percent, the same schedule applies to your reconstructive expenses.

Your insurance company may legally impose restrictions on payments it makes. You may be eligible for reconstruction or prostheses, for example, but not both. Even though your surgeon can perform some procedures in his office, your insurer may pay only if they are performed in a hospital or other surgical facility.

Your health insurance probably won't pay for procedures it considers "medically unnecessary." It might pay to exchange an implant if it ruptures, for example, but not because you want to switch from saline to silicone or would like a bigger size. Some insurance companies take the same view of nipple reconstruction, considering it an unnecessary cosmetic procedure. You may have to keep after them, and provide a letter from your doctor, to receive payment for this procedure.

Unfortunately, many companies also consider prophylactic mastectomy as medically unnecessary. If your health insurer refuses to preauthorize your prophylactic mastectomy, ask your oncologist, surgeon and/or medical geneticist to write memos explaining your high-risk status and supporting your decision to remove your breasts. Some insurers initially refuse to cover prophylactic surgery until they are convinced it may save the cost of dealing with future breast cancer. It's a cold way to view your health, but sometimes it's necessary to get the coverage you deserve.

The cost of reconstruction. If you're paying out-of-pocket for all or a portion of your reconstruction bill, you'll want to know what the process will cost. Your surgeon may require a deposit—50 percent of the total cost is typical—before your scheduled operation. Rates vary regionally and between physicians. Depending on the surgeon, operating facility, and reconstructive procedure, total cost may range from $10,000 to $40,000.

The following costs reflect fees for ASPS member surgeons in 2001. Additional costs for the general surgeon (who does the mastectomy), anesthesiologist, pathologist, operating room, and hospital room are not included in these figures.

Average Fees for Breast Reconstruction (2001)

- $2,841 for an implant.
- $3,413 for a tissue expander.
- $5,656 for a *latissimus dorsi* tissue flap.*
- $7,088 for an attached TRAM flap.**
- $9,315 for a free flap procedure. **

A tissue flap taken from the back (explained in Chapter 12).
**Tissue flaps taken from the abdomen (explained in Chapter 11).*

Source: ASPS member surgeons

Where to find help. If you have a question or problem with your insurance claim, start with the company's Customer Service Department. Hopefully, everything will go smoothly. Sometimes, that's not the case. Representatives often have training for only basic issues. They may not be able to tell you exactly what your coverage is, or advise you to submit a claim after the fact. That's bad advice you may later regret. You may get a different answer every time you call. If the information you need isn't provided in your plan document, request a written copy of the coverage from your insurer. Follow up until you receive it. Don't be shy about escalating to get your questions answered. Always document the date of the conversation, the name of the person who gave you the information and what you were told.

What to ask. Here's a sample list of the type of issues you should discuss with your insurance company before your reconstruction:

Questions for Your Health Insurance Company

- What reconstructive procedures are covered?
- Is immediate reconstruction covered?
- Will you pay for delayed reconstruction? If so, for what period of time after my mastectomy?
- Is there a limit to the amount of coverage provided?
- Am I limited to in-network surgeons and services? If I travel to another to another surgeon who specializes in a particular technique not available within your network, what expenses will be covered?
- Is my hospital stay covered? If so, for how many days?
- Under what conditions will you pay if I need additional procedures to correct problems related to my reconstruction?
- For what costs, if any, am I responsible?
- Will all bills be paid directly to providers or will I be reimbursed?

Your responsibility. Deal proactively with your insurance company to avoid problems down the road. Before your surgery, check your benefits handbook or plan document to determine what is covered. Call the insurance company's Customer Service Department if you need further clarification. If your plan requires preauthorization before any services are provided, be sure to comply. Don't take any payment for granted.

Ultimately, you're responsible for payment; you'll be asked to sign a form to that effect before surgery. If you receive an invoice in error, check to see if your insurance has been billed. Sometimes billing offices forget to invoice insurance companies or don't have the right information. Health insurers process thousand of claims and are often slow in paying; many billing offices expect you to call and check on payment. You may continue to receive bills every 30 days until payment is received. Don't panic and don't write a check. Contact your insurance company if your claim isn't paid within 90 days of the billing date. Keep your doctor's billing representative in the loop—she's used to dealing with insurance companies and is your best advocate.

If your claim is denied. Having written preauthorization eliminates a lot of headaches—and potential bills. Don't give up if your insurance company refuses your claim. First, determine why it was denied. Sometimes the wrong surgical code or vague language is the culprit. Then speak with the billing personnel at your hospital or doctor's office. If the claim is still denied, speak with a supervisor in your employer's Human Resources Department or submit an appeal (your benefits handbook or insurance carrier can explain the process). When pressed, many companies reverse their initial denials.

If you feel you're being treated unfairly or illegally, contact your state legislator or insurance oversight agency (usually the Insurance Commission, Department of Insurance, or the Health and Welfare Department). You can review a copy of your state's health insurance consumer guide at www.healthinsuranceinfo.net.

When you don't have health insurance. If you don't have insurance, ask your doctor's billing office if you can establish a payment plan. You'll have to deal with the hospital, anesthesiologist, pathologist, and other service providers separately. If you can't afford to pay, you may be eligible for state or federal programs for low-income and uninsured women. Most breast cancer financial aid doesn't extend to reconstruction, but it may be worth a call to your nearby ACS office to see if local aid is available. Another option is to contact a local medical center or teaching facility to see if they provide discounted services.

Tax deductible expenses. The IRS allows you to deduct out-of-pocket medical expenses in excess of 7.5 percent of your adjusted gross income from your income tax (line 33, Form 1040). You're allowed to deduct costs associated with your breast cancer and reconstruction, and all other health-related expenses you pay during the tax year, including co-payments and deductibles; braces for your kids; health care premiums; dental exams and procedures; eye exams, contact lenses, and eyeglasses; and books, magazines, or other materials related to your treatment (including this book). Travel costs, including mileage to and from the doctor or hospital, are also deductible. You may not deduct expenses for which you are reimbursed.

Keep receipts for everything you paid. If your surgeon recommends a special bra, camisole or other garment, ask for a prescription, so you'll have a written record. Tax laws change frequently. Check with your tax professional or see IRS Publication 502 for a complete list of deductible expenses.

> *My insurance company was great. My benefits manual outlined how mastectomy and reconstruction were covered. I never even saw a bill, so I assume everything was paid.* – Dawn

> *My managed care group didn't include any plastic surgeons. I had to look for one who was willing to negotiate a special contract. No one would accept the low payment the health company offered, so I ended up paying for the surgery myself.* – Paula

The Decision Roadmap

If you decide to have reconstruction, you'll need to make four key decisions regarding your procedure. As you come to understand more about your options, you'll have the information you need to make each one.

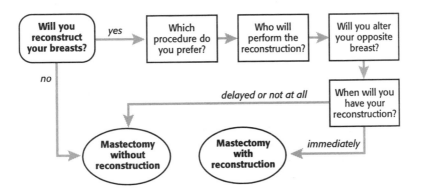

Chapter 8

Taming the Wild Ride

Trouble is a part of life,
and if you don't share it,
you don't give the person who loves you
a chance to love you enough.

— Dinah Shore

Dealing with the loss of your breast drops you smack in the front row of an emotional roller coaster. Even after you make the decision to have your breast reconstructed, you may still have doubts about the procedure. How will your new breast look? Is there some side effect of reconstruction you haven't discovered? Will your cancer come back? It's not unusual to have these feelings. Experts say shock, denial, anger, and depression typically come before acceptance. Meanwhile life goes on around you: there are dogs to feed, kids to be hugged, work to be done, and a house to manage.

Reflect and Accept

It takes time to get used to the idea of losing a breast. Sometimes it takes a lot of tears, too. Thoroughly researching reconstruction and knowing what to expect should provide some peace of mind and restore a measure of your confidence.

Don't hide from your feelings. Grief and angst come in all sizes. Some women are emotional Arnold Schwarzeneggers; they seem to take mastectomy and reconstruction in stride with "I-don't-have-time-for-cancer" attitudes. Others find it impossible to regain any sense of the normal during treatment and reconstruction. It's okay—and healthy— to react in a way that's natural for you. At some point, though, you'll get tired of being angry, tired of being sad, and tired of having your life put on hold. The best possible therapy is to acknowledge your feelings and let 'em rip. Then dust off your emotional self and move forward.

Create an outlet for your emotions. Don't get caught in a downward spiral of adverse emotions. Deal with your feelings before they begin controlling your life. Talk to your partner, a trusted friend, a member of the clergy, or support group members. Writing is also therapeutic. Try your hand at poetry or journaling during your breast cancer and reconstruction experience, letting the words flow freely onto the paper or computer screen.

Turn off the negative self-talk. It happens to the best of us: sooner or later those negative thoughts creep into our consciousness. When you catch yourself thinking negatively, replace your thoughts with positive affirmations. Focus on your post-reconstruction life. Consider the control reconstruction gives you, instead of dwelling on the loss from mastectomy.

Alone in my house, I cried all day. I was thankful for reconstruction, but I just couldn't come to grips with the reality of losing my breasts. My husband became so frustrated when he couldn't comfort me, he broke down and cried too. That was the day I decided I was done crying. – Kathy

Keep your hands and mind busy. Even the most proficient multitasker can't think about reconstruction when her mind is otherwise occupied. Begin a new family project. Garden, paint, or create in the kitchen. Do what you would normally do. Better yet, if you can spare the time, get involved helping others—there's no better way to get your mind off your own troubles than by helping someone else. Volunteer at your library, YWCA, or breast cancer center. Engage your mind and put your own reconstruction issues on the back burner for awhile each day.

Reprioritize. Actor Michael J. Fox once said, "Illness forces you to get rid of the clutter in your life to make room for the priorities." He was referring to his own fight against Parkinson's Disease, but his words ring true for any life-altering experience. Figure out what's important in your life and move those things to the top of your priority list. Don't feel guilty about items that float to the bottom and don't get done.

Keep your breast cancer and reconstruction in perspective. No one likes hearing "it could be worse," but in most cases, it's true. Regain perspective and hang on to it as much as possible. Remind yourself it's easier to replace a breast than an eye, leg, arm, or other functional part of your body. It is a bit of a cliché, but cancer *does* change your perspective. Treatment and reconstruction offer positives for those who are open to them. Learn—or re-learn—to appreciate life and all it offers. Separate the nickel-and-dime issues, like getting stuck in traffic or burning the toast, from the truly serious.

> *When my oncologist told me I needed a mastectomy, I screamed at him, "Why me, why me!" He calmly looked at me and said there were at least three or four patients in his waiting room who would change places with me in an instant.*
> – Patty

Keep your goals in sight. We all need something to look forward to, especially during trying times. Keep visual reminders of your post-reconstruction goals at hand. Hang pre-breast cancer photos of yourself on the refrigerator to remind yourself you'll once again look just fine in your favorite blouse or sweater. Stick a travel brochure of your planned post-reconstruction vacation to the mirror or prop it up on your desk.

Don't forget to laugh. Cancer and reconstruction certainly aren't funny, but we can always find humor if we look hard enough. Laughter is powerful medicine. It releases endorphins, sending feel-good messages from the brain throughout the body. Studies suggest laughter boosts the immune system and reduces pain. One little chuckle or a rollicking belly laugh releases a lot of tension. Have you ever noticed how quickly kids rebound from sadness? It may have everything to do with laughter. Children laugh about 400 times a day; adults, just 25. Find ways to laugh each day. The Cancer Club (800-586-9062 or www.cancerclub.com) has books, newsletters, and other items to tickle your funny bone and help you see the lighter side of treatment and reconstruction.

Adjust Your Attitude

It's often said that cancer is a journey. Sometimes we don't realize that until we reach the end of the process and look back. If only hindsight arrived a little sooner! If you can view reconstruction that way—as an odyssey with an outcome—you'll fare better. When you're uncomfortable, uneasy, or tired of the reconstruction ordeal, remember it isn't a life sentence. It's a finite experience with a beginning, a middle, and an end.

You won't ever forget your breast cancer or reconstruction. But you will be fine. Your emotional and physical scars will heal, and you'll return to a life without surgeons, weird sleeping positions, or checking your breasts throughout the day.

Finding Inspiration

We all have our own sources of inspiration. Family, friends, and sometimes, faith give us strength when we most need it. A touching poem, a special quotation, or a meaningful song lyric can diffuse our uneasiness. Breast cancer gives you the opportunity to find new inspiration. Find solace with members of a support group. Remind yourself how many people care about you: reread all the cards, letters, and e-mails you receive from well-wishers. Perhaps you'll find comfort and resolve in the Alcoholics Anonymous Serenity Prayer—if you didn't know otherwise, you might think it was written about breast reconstruction:

> *God, grant me the serenity to accept the things I cannot change; the courage to change the things I can; and the wisdom to know the difference.*

If you're looking for stories of courage and confidence, they're as close as your local ACS branch or breast cancer center. Your library and bookstore shelves are also crammed with personal stories of men and women who have gone through the same emotional upheaval you're experiencing, and much more. Here are three exceptional examples:

- *It's Not about the Bike—My Journey Back to Life* is champion cyclist Lance Armstrong's story about his fight with testicular cancer. Given only a slim chance of survival at age 25, he beat his cancer and went on to win an unprecedented fourth Tour de France. Although this story isn't about breast cancer, Armstrong's book is the ultimate inspiration for confronting disease and learning from the experience.

- *Ice Bound: A Doctor's Incredible Battle for Survival at the South Pole* describes how Dr. Jeri Neilsen self-biopsied a lump in her breast and administered her own chemotherapy while stranded at an arctic research station. Dr. Neilsen shares the emotional turmoil and intense introspection she experienced during her breast cancer.

- *Spinning Straw into Gold* by psychotherapist and breast cancer survivor Ronnie Kaye explains how to deal with the emotional side effects of breast cancer.

Each time I entered the hospital for a blood test, my hands began to shake and a feeling of dread came over me. I had to find a more positive perspective to get through my reconstruction. I began to consider hospitals and doctors as places and people who did things for me rather than to me. I started to consider reconstruction as the process that would put me back on the road to wholeness.
– Dora

You're Not Alone

Breast cancer and reconstruction can be very tough roads to walk alone. No one can have the surgery for you. No one can shorten your recovery or feel your pain. But you don't have to go it alone. If you let them, friends and family will rally to your side, providing endless love and strength to see you through the tough times and share the good times.

Recruit loved ones to care for your children, pets, and home while you're recovering. When friends ask how they can help, suggest they run errands, schedule a meal brigade or drive you to doctor appointments. Ask a friend to help you sort through information about reconstructive choices.

Never underestimate the power and support of those who care about you—including total strangers. No matter where you are, there's a huge sisterhood of breast cancer survivors with reconstruction experience who are waiting to lend an ear. They've been there. They can relate to what you're feeling better than anyone else. Ask your plastic surgeon for a referral to a previous patient who has had the same procedure. Call your local ACS or breast health center to join in a support group. Log on to the FORCE discussion group mentioned in Chapter 7 to get answers to your questions and calm your fears. Don't be afraid to say "not now" if you're not up to a visit or telephone call. It's good to have time to yourself, to reflect, accept, and just be.

Talking about Your Reconstruction

A generation ago, cancer was a mysterious disease shrouded in secrecy and shame. Today, most people know someone with breast cancer. Many women speak openly about their treatment, reconstruction, and recovery. Your own comfort level will dictate how much detail you share, and with whom. Some women feel comfortable telling only their closest family and friends about reconstruction, preferring not to advertise their new breasts. Others happily share every detail with anyone who will listen.

The wonderful and the weird. Your behavior sets the tone for how most people react. If you feel uncomfortable talking about reconstruction, others will too. Talking openly with friends and family will help them feel more at ease and encourage dialogue.

While most people are sensitive and compassionate about breast cancer and reconstruction, be prepared. People say and do the weirdest things. Friends may not be able to look you in the eye without crying. You may find yourself comforting them, instead of the other way around. Others may be embarrassed or struggle for the right thing to say. Some may be unable to accept the fact that you're fine, even after your recovery. They'll continue to view you as someone who is ill, even.long after you're back to your normal routine. Each time they see you, they ask in a soft, sad voice, "How are you?"

People often can't resist sharing their own breast cancer stories and will give you all the details of their friend's diagnosis and treatment. Don't be surprised if some folks can't seem to draw their eyes away from your chest. Many are quite curious about mastectomy and reconstruction; when they realize they are talking to your chest, they may become terribly embarrassed. They're all trying to help, in their own way. Just take a deep breath and realize they mean no harm.

Sometimes what people say doesn't really reflect their feelings. Don't be offended or hurt if the most insensitive words fly right out of people's mouths, like the following comments actually spoken to reconstruction patients:

Upon declining a lunch invitation:	"Oh, I guess you just don't want to be seen in public."
Regarding reconstruction:	"A friend at work had reconstruction two years ago and she's still in pain."
	"You're not considering implants, are you?"
About breast cancer:	"My aunt had breast cancer, too, and she died."

When your partner has a problem. Reconstruction patients often fear how their partners will react to their new breast. If your spouse or partner is supportive, you are truly blessed. Most women find their partners to be constant sources of reassurance, loving them for who they are, instead of what's on their chest. Ideally, your partner will accompany you to doctor's visits and participate fully in your research about reconstruction. If you and your partner share a strong

My four-year old had already seen me bald and sick after chemotherapy, so when I told him I was going back to the hospital for a few days to get better, he didn't even blink.
– Christine

Our puppy had to have surgery after he swallowed pillow stuffing. I explained Mommy's boobs had a type of stuffing that could make me sick, so a nice doctor was going to replace the bad stuffing with the good stuffing. I would be in the hospital, as our puppy had, and then would come home and soon be all better. I gave each of my children a teddy bear I said was filled with "Mommy love" that would never run out. Whenever I couldn't hug them, they could cuddle the bears and it would be like me giving them a big squeeze. – Cathy

relationship before breast cancer, you'll likely have the support you need during mastectomy and reconstruction. If your relationship was already weak, your treatment and reconstruction can bring you closer together—or drive you farther apart.

Some partners are scared silly by the thought of cancer and surgery, but hesitant to discuss their feelings. Others react with denial, refusing to acknowledge your cancer and reconstruction. Some—hopefully few—may wonder what the big deal is if you're able to have your breast recreated.

The more you can discuss reconstruction openly and honestly, the better your chance of getting through it together. Engage your partner's participation. Consider his or her opinion regarding different procedures. If it's difficult for the two of you to speak about reconstruction, encourage your partner to talk with a friend or medical expert, or attend breast cancer support groups with you. You need physical and emotional support during your reconstruction and recovery. If you don't find it at home, look to other resources mentioned throughout this book.

Talking with your kids. Your breast cancer and reconstruction affect your entire family. Most women feel it is better to tell children about reconstruction instead of keeping it a secret. Children know when something is wrong, even if they don't know what it is. They want to be reassured their world will remain unchanged. Tailor your explanations to each child's personality and level of understanding. Kids process information differently. Some ask lots of questions. Others aren't interested. Your demeanor influences their reaction. If they see you're okay, they'll be okay.

Keep it simple for little ones. Don't go overboard with details. If they don't already know about your breast cancer and treatment, reassure them you're not ill because of anything they did. Some women prefer to avoid using the word "sick," which may frighten children.

Maintain your child's sense of security. Let them know you'll be alright. Keep their routines as normal as possible. Explain you won't be able to pick them up for a few days (or more), and they must be careful not to jump on you. If you're emotional around your children, explain that Mommy is sad or angry or afraid, but not because of them.

Older children and teens will want to know more. They may feel frightened or threatened if they sense reconstruction is a taboo topic. Reassure them you'll be fine, and that your reconstruction is a way to help restore your breast after mastectomy. Let them know how they can help during your recovery.

Talking to people at work. Your relationship with your co-workers will dictate how much you do or don't tell them about your treatment and reconstruction. Many women consider their co-workers as an extended family, while others prefer not to draw attention to themselves or be treated differently.

You may have already discussed your treatment with your boss or supervisor. If you're uncomfortable talking about your reconstruction, you need to at least inform him of your need for time off for health reasons—how much you tell him is up to you. At the very minimum, he'll need to know how long you'll be away from work and any restrictions on your return:

"It's a three-step procedure over the next nine months."

"I'll be out for about four weeks; then I'll be back without restrictions."

"I'll return in six weeks, but I won't be able to lift anything over five or six pounds for another three to four weeks."

You'll also need to discuss time off for additional doctor appointments, particularly if you'll be having tissue expansion.

Reconstructive Procedures

Chapter 9

Breast Implants

We could never learn to be brave and patient
if there were only joy in the world.
– Helen Keller

Before surgeons perfected tissue flap surgery, implants were the only method of reconstructing breasts after mastectomy. Used for more than 40 years, implants now account for about half of all breast reconstructions.

Compared to tissue flap procedures, implant surgery is shorter, requires less skill, and leaves fewer scars. It's also less costly. Recovery from surgery is faster, but the entire reconstruction process takes longer to complete.

While most women are happy with their implants, there are downsides. With unilateral reconstruction, it can be difficult to match your natural breast without additional surgery, because implants can't be shaped and sculpted like living tissue. Your implanted breast won't droop or reflect weight changes like your opposite breast, so you may become asymmetrical over time. Unlike living tissue, implants are devices: they are susceptible to complications, and sooner or later must be replaced.

Saline or Silicone

Breast implants are filled with saline (sterile saltwater) or silicone gel. You may have heard about implants filled with soybean oil or covered with polyurethane foam. These are no longer available.

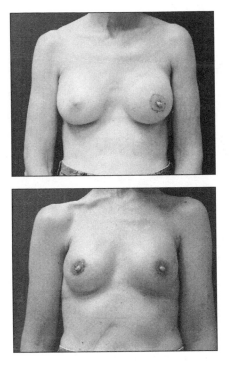

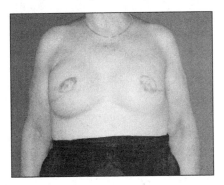

Unilateral reconstruction of left breast (left), immediate bilateral reconstruction after skin-sparing mastectomies (bottom left), and delayed bilateral reconstruction (bottom right).

Saline implants are filled in the operating room just before they are used. The surgeon injects a saltwater solution directly into a valve on top of the implant or via a filler tube which is removed once the implant reaches the desired size. Silicone implants are filled by the manufacturer.

A breast reconstructed with a saline implant is firm, like a water balloon filled to capacity. It doesn't have the resilience and bounce of silicone gel, which feels and moves more like your own breast. If you're opposed to having silicone in your body, you should know that all implants, including those filled with saline, have outer shells of silicone elastomer, a thin medical-grade rubber. Virtually everyone has some exposure to silicone, because it's widely used in cosmetics, fabrics, lotions, adhesives, lubricants, gum, tires, and thousands of other products we use every day. Medical grade silicone is used in pharmaceutical products and medical devices, including heart shunts, pacemakers, and artificial limbs.

Ask your surgeon for samples of saline and silicone implants, so you can touch them and compare how they feel. He can put you in contact with other patients who have had implant reconstruction; you can hear what they have to say. Some may even be willing to give you a peek or a poke at their results.

Defining your new shape. Your surgeon selects a round or contoured implant with a diameter to match your chest. Round implants are used more frequently in reconstruction. Contoured or teardrop-shaped implants provide more projection than round models, although placing a contoured implant under the muscle causes it to assume a rounder, flatter shape. Your chest structure, the amount of muscle, and the elasticity of your breast skin influence the shape of your new breast as much, if not more, than the type of implant used.

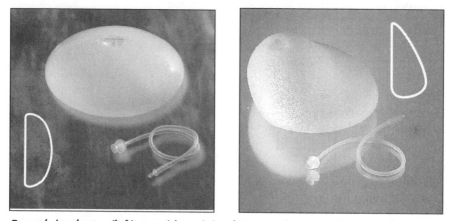

Round implants (left) provide minimal to moderate projection. Contoured implants (right) provide maximum projection, but not all women have the chest structure to accommodate them.

Older style implants always had smooth surfaces. Some models are now textured to reduce the chance of hard scar tissue adhering to the implant and distorting its shape. However, complications occur more frequently with textured implants.

Reconstruction by Type of Implant

TYPE	PERCENT OF TOTAL
Textured saline	46
Smooth saline	29
Textured silicone gel	11
Smooth silicone gel	9
Permanent expander	4

Total is less than 100% due to rounding.

Source: ASPS member surgeons (2000)

The question of size. Discussing implant size isn't as easy as saying, "Make me a 36B." Because most women's bras don't fit their breasts correctly, bra size is an unreliable measurement. Nor are there industry standards when it comes to bra size. Buy size 36B bras from three different companies and you'll likely get three different fits.

Implant size is defined by volume measured in cubic centimeters (cc).

    60 cc = 2 ounces (4 tablespoons)
    120 cc = 4 ounces (1/2 cup)
    240 cc = 8 ounces (1 cup)
    480 cc = 16 ounces (2 cups)

Generally, it takes about 190 cc for one bra cup size. A B-cup breast, for example, requires an implant of about 380 cc.

If you're having unilateral reconstruction, your surgeon will choose an implant that matches the size and shape of your opposite breast as closely as possible. With bilateral reconstruction, you have a somewhat clean slate. You may want to restore your pre-mastectomy breast size, or choose smaller or bigger breasts. If you're unsure how to describe what you want, provide a photo for your surgeon. Look through underwear and swimsuit catalogs, or even men's magazines for ideas. It also helps to provide photos of what you consider to be too small and too large.

Selecting an implant of the right dimension and volume is critical to good results: an implant too small won't give you the cleavage you want and may cause the breast skin to wrinkle or ripple. An implant too large may extend beyond the chest pocket and you may be able to feel or see the edges.

Are They Safe?

Breast implants have been around in one form or another for decades. After World War II, Japanese prostitutes thought if they could make their breasts bigger, American soldiers might find them more attractive. The women tried injecting wax, peanut butter, mineral oil, and industrial-grade liquid silicone into their breasts. None of these methods worked, and the silicone proved to be quite dangerous. Some people still consider silicone implants dangerous, although the evidence is conflicting. For each report hyping the dangers of silicone implants, there's another supporting their safety.

The first silicone implants were developed in 1961 by two plastic surgeons and the Dow Corning Corporation. Saline implants were introduced four years later, and the breast augmentation boom began. By the 1970s, several manufacturers were mass-producing implants to meet rapidly growing demand. By the time the Food and Drug Administration (FDA) actually began regulating implants in 1976, thousands of women already had them.

In 1990, a woman sued Dow Corning, claiming the firm's silicone implants caused her autoimmune disease. Subsequently, more than 9,000 similar individual and class action suits were filed against Dow and other implant manufacturers. The media had a field day. Surgeons and health organizations were caught between a rock and a hard place. Although silicone implants had been used for almost 30 years without controversy or reports of significant health problems, neither saline nor silicone models had ever been evaluated for long-term safety.

The FDA banned the use of silicone implants for cosmetic purposes in 1992, until definitive evidence could prove they were safe. The FDA did, however, approve use of the devices to replace existing silicone implants or repair congenital defects. It also approved the implants for breast reconstruction for women who agreed to be followed in a long-term study. That same year, Dow Corning filed for bankruptcy. Today, just two manufacturers, Inamed Aesthetics, formerly McGhan Medical Corporation, (800-862-4426 or www.inamed.com) and Mentor Corporation (800-525-0245 or www.mentorcorp.com), provide most of the implants used in the United States. Dow and other implant companies established a joint $4 billion compensation package in 1994.

In 1997, the FDA chartered the Institute of Medicine (IOM) to conduct an independent review of all past and ongoing scientific research regarding the safety of silicone breast implants. The IOM found no evidence linking implants to cancer, connective tissue disorders, autoimmune diseases, or other significant health problems. Subsequent studies in the United States, including those by the Mayo Clinic and Harvard, Canada, and Europe found no link between silicone implants and disease.

The IOM, however, did note that both saline and silicone implants frequently develop complications, which often require additional medical intervention, including surgery. You can read a summary of the IOM's findings in *Information for Women about the Safety of Silicone Breast Implants*, available from Y-ME National Breast Cancer Organization (800-221-2141 or www.yme.org). As of this writing, the ban on silicone implants remains in place. FDA guidelines may change as more information about the safety of silicone implants becomes available. In 2000, the FDA approved the use of saline implants—35 years after they were first used. Contact the FDA (888-463-6332 or www.fda.gov/cdrh/breastimplants/) for a copy of *The Breast Implant Consumer Handbook* and silicone implant study data.

Safety isn't the only issue. Statistics are one thing; experience is quite another. While most women are satisfied with their implant reconstruction, those who aren't say related problems can range from annoying to devastating. The IOM agreed, finding implants to be safe, but noting three negative findings:

- Frequent local (confined to the breast) problems.

- The need to replace implants sooner or later.

- Medical intervention, including surgery, is required to address problems.

These problems and others are discussed later in this chapter.

Federal law requires all women who have implant surgery be given a copy of the product information sheet that comes with each device. Ask for it if your surgeon doesn't provide a copy. Read the information carefully. Consider the advantages and disadvantages of both silicone and saline implants before you decide how your reconstruction will be done.

Implant Procedures

Reconstruction is never a one-step process. First the breast mound is created, then a separate procedure creates the nipple and areola. Most implant procedures involve three stages:

1. Expanding the skin.

2. Placing the implant.

3. Recreating the nipple and areola.

Most immediate and all delayed reconstructions begin with tissue expansion, because after mastectomy there is usually not enough breast skin to cover an implant of the desired size. Think of it this way: if you have a bag that holds a pound of rice, and you cut a portion of the fabric away, then sew the edges together, you've reduced the volume somewhat. It's the same after mastectomy. The remaining breast skin can hold only a somewhat smaller breast—just how much smaller depends on the amount of skin you have before your mastectomy and how much is removed.

Initially, a temporary implant called a tissue expander is placed under the muscle. As it is gradually inflated with saline over several weeks, the expander stretches the breast skin, similar to the way a pregnant woman's stomach skin expands.

The pocket procedure. The first step in implant surgery is creating a pocket under the *pectoralis major* muscle to hold the expander.

This muscle lies between the skin and the ribs. Creating a pocket is not difficult, since only the ends of the muscle are attached to the chest wall. The bulk of the muscle slides freely over the ribs as you move your arms and shoulders. Working through the mastectomy incision, the surgeon lifts the muscle and shapes the pocket. The pocket must be just the right size—not too big or the implant will move around; not too small or the implant will be too firm or distorted.

Implant Info	
Surgery	1-2 hours
Hospital stay	
immediate	1-2 days
delayed	overnight
Back to daily activities	2-3 weeks
Back to sports and strenuous activities	4-6 weeks

After the expander is tested for leaks, it is emptied and placed into the pocket—an empty expander allows for a smaller incision. The surgeon adds 60 to 100 cc of saline and closes the fill valve on the top of the expander. He sutures the muscle edges over the expander and places a surgical drain at the site. He closes the incision with dissolvable stitches and surgical tape. Finally, he places a surgical bra or compression garment (some look like elastic tube tops) over your breasts. This will stay in place until the surgeon removes it in his office in a few days. The operation takes about an hour for each breast.

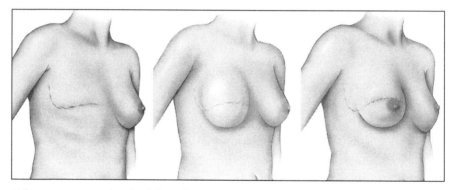

When reconstruction is delayed, a scar remains across the chest (left). Implant reconstruction begins by creating a breast mound with a tissue expander (center). Adding the nipple and areola completes the reconstruction. The mastectomy scar is visible across breast (right) but eventually fades.

When the expander is fully inflated, and the pocket is stretched enough to hold the implant, the expanded breast must settle for two to three months. Then a second, shorter operation is performed to replace the expander with a fixed-volume implant. The nipple and areola are created two or three months later, after the breast mound drops into its final position.

Timeline: tissue expander with fixed-volume implant (6-10 months)

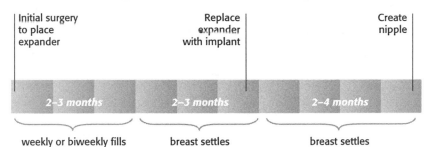

Initial surgery to place expander

Replace expander with implant

Create nipple

2-3 months | 2-3 months | 2-4 months

weekly or biweekly fills | breast settles | breast settles

Save-a-step reconstructions. If you prefer a small breast after mastectomy, you may be able to skip the exchange surgery by using a hybrid expander/implant. It has a silicone shell surrounding two inner layers: an outer layer of silicone gel over an inner layer of saline. The saline portion of the implant is gradually filled and adjusted like a tissue expander, while the silicone provides a more natural feel. When fully expanded to the desired size, the hybrid is sealed and remains in place, eliminating the need for exchange surgery.

Timeline: hybrid expander/implant (4-7 months)

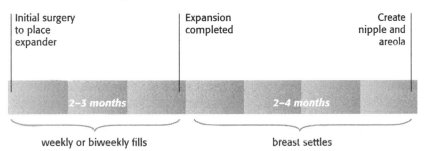

Initial surgery to place expander

Expansion completed

Create nipple and areola

2-3 months | 2-4 months

weekly or biweekly fills | breast settles

If you schedule immediate reconstruction and have sufficient breast skin, expansion may not be necessary. Your surgeon can reconstruct your breast with a small fixed-volume implant. He performs the same pocket procedure described for expanders. An empty implant is placed into the pocket, then filled with saline. Silicone implants are placed at full volume and require longer incisions.

Some implants are adjustable, allowing the surgeon to fine-tune breast size after surgery. If, after living with your implants for a while, you'd like to be a bit smaller, your surgeon can remove some of the saline. If you want to be somewhat larger, he can add saline. When you're happy with the size, the filler port is removed. While both hybrid and fixed-volume implants eliminate the exchange operation, additional surgery may be needed to reshape or reposition the reconstructed breast.

Timeline: fixed-volume implant (3-4 months)

Initial surgery
to place
implant

Create
nipple and
areola

3–4 months

breast settles

Recovery

If you have immediate implant reconstruction after your mastectomy, you'll stay in the hospital for a day or two. If your reconstruction is delayed, you may go home the same day or stay overnight. Your breast area will be numb. It may feel heavy or ache for a few days, more from cutting into the muscle than the mastectomy. If your lymph nodes were removed during your surgery, you may be numb or sore under your arm. Any discomfort is usually controlled by pain medication.

You'll be encouraged to get up and begin walking the day after your surgery. You should take progressively longer walks each day. After your operation, you'll be able to carefully lift your arms to wash your face and brush your teeth. It will take another week or so before you can lift them over your head. You'll be very tired and sore for a couple of weeks, but your strength will slowly return. Each day you'll spend more time awake and less time napping. Your surgeon will show you how to properly exercise your upper body after surgery to regain full mobility and range of motion. Chapter 18 also provides helpful exercises.

Living with implants. They're perky and they stay that way. Implants, especially saline models, don't bounce or jiggle much when you move or flop to the side when you lie on your back. When someone hugs you they feel quite firm. Silicone implants feel and move more like a natural breast. Some women, however, say their silicone implants always feel cold.

Bras are optional with implants. You certainly won't need to wear one, but many women enjoy wearing pretty lingerie after reconstruction. You might need a different size bra than you're used to, because your new breast may be a different shape or size than your pre-mastectomy breast. You may be limited to wearing seamless stretch bras if your breast doesn't have enough projection to fill a regular bra. If you have unilateral implant reconstruction, your new breast may not match the exact shape, size, or projection as your opposite breast.

Before surgery, you may wonder if you'll always be conscious of your implants. Will they ever feel a part of you, as your natural breasts did? At first, you'll be very aware of your implanted breast. It will feel heavy. You'll feel it shift in the pocket when you stretch or lift. This isn't painful, but it can feel odd until you become accustomed to it. If you flex your chest muscle, your implanted breast will move. After a few months, your implants will become somewhat softer, feel more natural, and drop a little on your chest. You will get used to them in time.

Are Implants Right for You?

More than two million women in the United States have implants, but they're not right for everyone. Implant surgery is not advised for women who have lupus, scleroderma, other autoimmune diseases, or health conditions that interfere with healing or blood clotting. Your reconstruction must be delayed until infection anywhere in your body is treated and resolved. Implant reconstruction is a good option for women who:

- Aren't opposed to having silicone or saline in their bodies.

- Don't mind going through the lengthy expansion process.

- Are willing to surgically alter their opposite breast for symmetry.

- Have enough muscle and overlying tissue to accommodate an expander or an implant.

Radiation and implants. The IOM study confirmed radiation doesn't harm implants, nor do implants interfere with radiation. Most surgeons agree, however, that radiation and implants are a poor combination. Radiation reduces blood circulation and elasticity in the skin and underlying tissue. The skin may not expand enough to accommodate an implant; it may squeeze the

My surgeon warned me about a poor result if we used an implant after radiation, but I didn't want to have flap surgery. He was right. The skin and muscle of my irradiated breast squeezes the implant, no matter how much saline is put in. It's smaller and harder than the other breast and has a big dent in one side.
– Angie

implant and distort its shape. It's not impossible to expand radiated skin, but it's difficult and often produces less-than-satisfactory results.

Although not ideal, better results may be achieved when the breast is expanded and reconstructed before radiation. A small study at Memorial Sloan Kettering Hospital found more than 80 percent of women who had radiation after implant reconstruction had good to excellent results. Eighty-two percent of the women said they would choose implant reconstruction again.

Potential Problems

Women either love or hate their implants. Most are quite satisfied with their implant reconstructions and say they would have the same surgery again, but many experience repeated problems. As stated in the IOM study, the real issue with implants is not a link to disease or serious health conditions, but the frequent need for medical intervention or surgery to repair problems with the implant itself. If you're considering implant reconstruction, carefully factor these potential complications into your decision-making process.

Implants don't last forever. Like washing machines, DVDs, and other manmade products, sooner or later implants wear out. The average lifespan of an implant is about seven to 10 years. There's no way to predict how long yours will last or if it will develop a problem. While some women have implants for years without complication, others have repeated problems that can only be fixed by removing and/or replacing the implant. Most women will have their implants replaced at least once and possibly more during their lifetimes. This risk of replacement increases as the implant ages.

A retrospective study of women with saline or silicone implant reconstruction between 1964 and 1991 found 20 percent (one in five) needed a corrective operation within one year. More than 33 percent (one in three) required surgery within five years. More recently, studies by Inamed and Mentor found 40 percent of women with saline implant reconstruction needed additional surgery within three years.

Replacing your implant. If your implant is removed for any reason, you're back to square one: what should you do with your now-absent breast? While most women replace their implants, others switch to tissue flaps to avoid future complications and additional replacement surgeries. Some take the opportunity to exchange silicone implants for saline or vice versa. If you decide not to reconstruct again, most of your breast skin will be removed and you'll have a slanting scar across your chest, as if you had a mastectomy without reconstruction.

Unless complications occur, it's not particularly difficult to replace an implant. The pocket is already there, so most of the work is done. The surgeon accesses the pocket through the earlier incision, removes the implant, and puts in a new one. Generally, replacing a saline implant can be done in an hour or so with minimal discomfort. The process can be much more involved when silicone leaks beyond the implant.

No matter how easy it is to replace an implant, the process can be emotionally devastating: you're happily living your post-cancer life when you must undergo more doctor visits and additional surgery to repair a problem with your new breast. Some women say it's like reliving their reconstruction all over again. Other women consider replacement surgery a price they're willing to pay. Either way, it's an important consideration to factor into your decision about which technique is best for you. In time, all implants age and weaken. Pacemakers must be replaced every 10 years or so. Perhaps that's the best way to view implants.

I want the easiest possible reconstruction. I don't mind if the implant must be exchanged in the future. It's required maintenance, like getting my car serviced every 30,000 miles. I can take a couple of days every few years to do that if I need to. Besides, maybe they'll have something better by then and I can trade up to a better model! – Belle

I can't bear the thought of going through more surgery every five or six or seven years. I'd rather have a flap reconstruction and get it over with once and for all. – Gisele

Following is a summary of the most common implant problems.

Ruptures and leaks. Some implants leak and deflate within a few months after surgery. Others last 15 to 20 years or more. It's difficult, if not impossible, to determine the rate of implant ruptures. The statistics are confusing and may be unreliable, because many ruptures are undetected. Newer implants are thought to be more reliable and leak less frequently. Ruptures and leaks can be caused by injury to the breast, normal aging of the implant, capsular contracture (see the following description), or other unknown reasons. There may be a small flaw in the shell or the surgeon may accidentally prick it while stitching the incision.

If a saline implant leaks, you'll know it, because your reconstructed breast will deflate like a balloon. The saline is safely absorbed by the body, but the implant must be replaced.

An MRI found a rupture in my silicone implant when it was six years old. My breast seemed fine. I didn't even know anything had happened. – Norene

After two implants ruptured in five years, I gave up. The last straw was when my saline implant leaked while I was on vacation. It was horrible. There I was on a beautiful tropical beach, wearing a big baggy shirt to cover my deflated breast. – Alma

When a silicone implant leaks, you might feel a hard knot, have pain or tingling, or notice a difference in the shape or size of your breast. Because the shell remains firm, you may have no symptoms at all.

If silicone does leak, it is often contained between the implant and the scar tissue around it. When this occurs, the implant and surrounding tissue must be removed, which can be very difficult. In some cases, an MRI or ultrasound detects lumps of gel beyond the breast or in the lymph nodes. It is desireable, but not always possible to remove silicone from the tissue. Some women develop gel bleed: although the implant doesn't leak, silicone leeches through the shell.

Two studies found ruptures in 51 to 55 percent of silicone implants placed prior to 1992. Twenty percent leaked into the surrounding tissue. Newer silicone implants may be safer—the gel is thicker and the shells are stronger. Many now have double lumen construction, with the added protection of a shell within a shell. Saline implants appear to have a better track record: six to nine percent deflate after reconstruction.

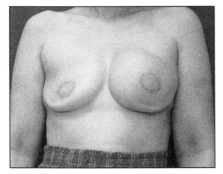

When a saline implant leaks, the water is safely absorbed by the body, but the implant must be removed and replaced.

Capsular contracture. After reconstruction, a capsule of scar tissue forms around the implant. This isn't unusual, and it isn't a health hazard. It's the body's natural reaction to foreign matter. This also occurs in patients who have pacemakers or artificial hips.

Capsular contracture occurs when the scar tissue tightens and squeezes the implant. It can be uncomfortable or painful, and distort the shape of the breast. Experts don't know why some women experience capsular contracture repeatedly, while others never have it. It can occur within a few months of reconstruction or years later. Placing the implant under the muscle, and gently massaging it and moving it around in the pocket may help limit the problem.

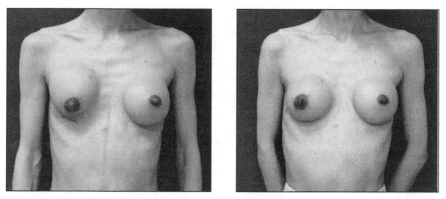

Capsular contracture occurs when scar tissue squeezes the implant and distorts the shape of the breast (left). Surgically removing the scar tissue and replacing the implant restores the reconstructed breast (right).

Capsular contracture is measured by the Baker Grade system. Mild capsular contracture (Grades I and II) may cause the breast to feel hard, but not enough to warrant any action. Severe cases (Grades III and IV) can be painful and distort the breast.

Grade I The breast is normally soft and looks natural.

Grade II The breast is a little firm but looks normal.

Grade III The breast is firm and is visibly distorted.

Grade IV The breast is hard, painful, and visibly distorted.

In years past, surgeons tried breaking the scar capsule by vigorously squeezing the implant, or striking it with the hand. These procedures are rarely used any longer and are not recommended by Inamed nor Mentor. It's sometimes possible to cut the scar tissue away from the implant in a *capsulectomy* procedure. In many cases, however, the implant must be removed, and if the patient wishes, replaced. There's no guarantee capsular contracture won't recur. The problem occurs 30 to 40 percent more frequently in women who have had radiation to the chest before implant reconstruction.

Infection. Only two to five percent of women develop infection after implant reconstruction, but it's a risk with any surgery. Symptoms include swelling, pain, fever, or redness in the breast. Infection is of particular concern with implants. If an infection doesn't respond to antibiotics, the implant may have to be removed to treat the chest pocket. A new implant can be placed when the infection has been resolved.

You'll be given antibiotics before and after your surgeries, and each time more saline is added to your expanders. As long as you have an implant, you should take antibiotics one or two days before and after any operation or invasive procedure, including dental work. This is a precautionary measure to prevent bacteria migrating in the blood or saliva from the mouth to the implant. Your surgeon can prescribe antibiotics when you need them.

Hematoma or seroma. Surgical drains usually prevent excess fluids form collecting in the breast, but sometimes a *hematoma,* a collection of blood, or a *seroma*, the watery portion of blood, pools at the mastectomy site. These fluids are usually absorbed by the body. In some instances, it may be necessary to place a surgical drain at the site for a few days.

Pain. While most women find their post-reconstruction pain gradually disappears, some experience breast pain or muscle spasms after their incisions have healed. Lingering pain is most often caused by infection, rupture, capsular contracture, or improperly sized implants. Infrequently, blood or fluid that collects around an implant can cause pain or other problems until it is drained. Chapter 19 discusses how to treat lingering pain.

Necrosis. Infrequently, a portion of tissue around the implant doesn't get enough blood and dies. This *necrosis* may be painful and delay healing. It occurs more often in women who are smokers, have circulatory problems, or those who have radiation or chemotherapy after their reconstruction.

Autoimmune disease. More than a decade after the landmark litigation against Dow Corning, the relationship between silicone implants and autoimmune disorders remains controversial. Although there is no hard evidence to the contrary and many doctors now consider silicone implants relatively safe, some experts still believe silicone can cause health problems for some women.

When a person has autoimmune disease, her immune system malfunctions and attacks itself. This can cause lupus, psoriasis, chronic fatigue syndrome, rheumatoid arthritis, and many other conditions.

A small percentage of women with silicone implants develop characteristics of these diseases. Some scientists explain that the number of women in this country with implants now exceeds two million, and that autoimmune problems will inevitably occur in a population of that size, with or without implants. In other words, autoimmune disease symptoms occur no more frequently in women with silicone implants than in those without the devices. Perhaps silicone acts as a catalyst in some women who may be predisposed to certain health conditions. In any case, if you currently suffer from arthritis, lupus, chronic fatigue, or other immune system weaknesses, you should probably choose a different type of reconstruction.

Cosmetic problems. Cosmetic imperfections can and do occur with implants. Sometimes the breast skin doesn't cover the implant adequately. Wrinkling and rippling may develop, more frequently in especially thin women and when textured saline implants are used. Some women may feel the edge of their implants or have asymmetry when compared to the opposite side. In rare cases, the implant may *extrude* or come through the skin. Contoured implants have been known to flip over in the pocket. All these problems can be corrected with additional surgery.

If the pocket is too large, an implant can move around or rotate. The solution is additional surgery to place a larger implant or reduce the size of the pocket. *Synmastia* occurs in bilateral reconstruction when the pockets on either side merge into one, eliminating the natural space between the breasts—the two breasts look as though they're joined in the middle. This happens when too much of the muscle is cut to create the pockets. Synmastia requires surgery to repair the muscle and replace the implants.

Product warranties. Both Mentor and Inamed warranty their products. Recipients are automatically covered by the manufacturers' standard warranties. The companies provide lifetime replacement of the implant and limited financial assistance to defray costs of future revision or replacement surgeries not covered by insurance. Extended warranties are also available.

Before your surgery, your doctor or his nurse should explain the terms of the warranty for your implant and give you a copy of the document. You can also access warranty information on the manufacturers' websites. Read the information carefully. Before you leave the hospital, the nurse will give you a card with the serial number of your implants. You'll need this information to activate your warranty.

Chapter 10

The Expander Experience

The way I see it, if you want the rainbow,
you gotta be willing to put up with the rain.

– Dolly Parton

Tissue expanders deserve an entire chapter to themselves, because if you decide to reconstruct your breasts with implants, most of the process will involve expanders. The expansion process can be awkward and uncomfortable. It can also be inconvenient; you'll be visiting your surgeon's office regularly for several weeks. Expanders and implants, however, provide a welcome alternative for women who prefer not to undergo the longer surgery or scarring of tissue flap reconstruction.

The expander's job is to stretch the skin and muscle to make room for the implant. Amazingly, the expansion process not only stretches, but creates new skin. Before reconstruction, your surgeon will measure your chest and select an expander of adequate size, diameter, and volume to create space for the size implant you want.

Getting Your Fill

During your initial reconstruction surgery, 60 to 100 cc of saline will be added to your empty expander. This will push the muscle forward, creating a little bulge. When you wake up, you'll have this starter breast mound, so you won't have to experience a completely flat chest. Within two or three weeks, or when your initial incision is healing well, you'll begin getting "fills" in your surgeon's office. As you lie flat, he'll use a magnetic device—like a mini version of a carpenter's stud finder—to locate the filler port just under your skin. You may be able to feel the port if you run your fingers over your breast skin. The surgeon will inject 50 to 120 cc of saline into the expander via the port. You shouldn't feel the needle, because your breast will be numb. Your chest will feel tight and full as the saline inflates the expander.

Each time saline is added, the expander stretches the muscle and surrounding skin a little more.

The surgeon will apply antibiotic ointment and sterile gauze, and you're done for the day. The entire procedure takes only 10 to 15 minutes for each side. You'll take antibiotics the day before and the day of the fill, to guard against infection. Every seven to 14 days, you'll go back for another fill. Most women are completely filled in six to eight weeks. Your own interval may be shorter or longer, depending on how much your skin must stretch and how well you tolerate the process. The chart below shows how the fill amount and frequency affects the length of time it takes to reach your expansion goal.

Sample Timetable for Fill Intervals				
BIWEEKLY FILL	*6 WEEKS*	*8 WEEKS*	*10 WEEKS*	*12 WEEKS*
60 cc	240	300	360	420
100 cc	360	460	560	660
140 cc	480	620		

Assumptions: Each fill adds the same amount of saline.
                    60 cc added at initial surgery.

Getting fills isn't usually painful, but it can be uncomfortable. As the expander stretches the muscle away from the ribcage, your chest may feel heavy or tender under your breast. The top of your breast will be softer and less uncomfortable, because those muscles aren't attached to ribs. You'll feel especially tight for several hours or a couple of days after each fill. Some women equate this to having braces on their teeth: just about the time they get used to their braces, the dentist tightens them, and they're uncomfortable all over again. The tightness will lessen in a few weeks when the muscle relaxes.

I heard about the horrible aches from expanders, but I didn't really feel too bad. I was a little tender after each fill, but that was about it. –Glenda

My doctor began filling my expanders with 120 cc every seven days. It was very uncomfortable for two or three days afterward. It felt like a metal band was crushing my ribs. I got in the habit of massaging my ribcage. I'd rub as I read, watched TV, even as I drove. It was temporary relief, but it helped. I finally asked my doctor to put in only 60 cc at a time. My expansion took longer, but it was more tolerable. – Lin

You'll continue getting fills until your expander is overfilled by about 10 percent. If your surgeon thinks your final implant size will be 500 cc, for example, he'll fill your expander to 550 cc. This ensures there will be more than enough skin to cover your implant. It also allows the implant to sit lower in the pocket, so your final breast won't sit unnaturally high on the chest.

Minimizing your discomfort. If you're uncomfortable during your expansion, Tylenol or other over-the-counter medication will help. Warmth may also provide temporary relief. Soak a towel or washcloth in very warm water, wring it out and hold it against your ribcage or under your expanding breast. If you're especially sore when you wake up, try a warm shower or some light stretching to warm up the muscles. Don't use a heating pad on the mastectomy site! With your post-mastectomy numbness, you won't feel the heat. You can easily burn without knowing it.

Gentle massage also relaxes the muscles and provides relief. Apply oil or lotion and rub along the side and front of the rib cage several times a day.

Speak up if you need smaller or less frequent fills. You'll be anxious to be done with the process, but take time to listen to your body. It will be worth it in the end. If your discomfort is severe, ask your surgeon to remove some saline. He can also give you a referral to a physical therapist, who can massage and relax the connective tissues in the chest.

Living in Limbo

Aside from the temporary discomfort, dressing during the expansion process can be a challenge. During unilateral expansion, a bra that fits your normal breast won't fit your expanding breast. You start out with a very small breast mound that grows progressively larger every few days. Early on in your expansion, you can wear a small prosthesis in your bra to even out your chest. As your breast mound grows larger, it will be higher and larger than your other breast. Camouflage seems to work well for most women during this stage. Try going without a bra, or wear vests, jackets, or other loose clothing.

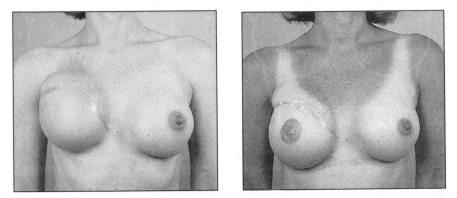

As your expander nears over-inflation, it may be larger and higher than your other breast (left). This will be corrected when the expander is exchanged for an implant. When completely finished, your new breast will be very similar to your opposite breast (right).

Light at the end of the tunnel. With each fill, you'll begin to see significant changes as your cleavage develops and the inframammary crease forms under your breast. You may be tired of the procedure and annoyed with the cosmetic disadvantages of expanders. Don't be disheartened if your reconstructed breast seems flatter, rounder, or higher than you expected. Hang in there if you feel lopsided or misshapen.

Remember, you're a work in progress. This is not the way your implanted breast will look. Expanders are temporary. Your discomfort is temporary. Don't be overly concerned with incisions that seem uneven or puckered. They'll be re-excised during your exchange surgery. Keep the end result in mind. In a few months your reconstruction will be over.

I was amazed that I had hardly any swelling or bruising, but I did have cleavage! At first, the expanders gave me a flat bulk, like a bodybuilder. My new breasts looked great when I looked down, but there wasn't much there from a side view. – Maureen

Exchange Surgery

Once your breast has expanded sufficiently and settled into the pocket, it's time to exchange it for an implant. This will provide welcome relief; the difference between expanders and implants is night and day.

I felt pretty good after my exchange surgery. I was a bit tired the first night, but then I felt just fine. It was nothing like the original operation. Having those expanders out gave me an overwhelming feeling of freedom. I spent the entire afternoon trying on clothes with my new breasts. — Madelyne

Oh, the joy of having those stupid expanders removed! Finally! No weird breasts under my collarbone. I could finally wear something other than baggy shirts. — Jessica

Exchange surgery is an outpatient procedure done in a hospital or surgical facility under general anesthesia. Once you're asleep, the surgeon re-opens your mastectomy scar and removes the expander. He then inserts your new implant into the pocket and shapes the skin around it. If necessary, your surgeon adjusts the pocket so the reconstructed breast is even with your opposite breast. If you're having bilateral reconstruction, he makes sure both breasts are positioned evenly.

A surgical drain is placed near the new breast and the incision is closed. Your chest is bound with a hospital dressing to discourage swelling. The exchange procedure takes about an hour or two. Compared to your initial operation, this operation is a snap. It's not as painful, and you'll recover in just a day or two.

Two or three days after the surgery, your surgeon will remove the hospital dressing. For the first time, you'll get a look at your new breast. It's a big improvement over the expanders, but it's still not the final product. Over the next few weeks, any swelling will subside and your implants will drop to a more normal position.

Potential Problems

Although most women don't have serious problems with expanders, complications can occur. The surgeon must first determine whether your breast site is healthy enough for expansion. Damage from radiation, poor post-mastectomy healing, insufficient blood flow to the skin, or other problems may postpone or preclude using expanders. If excess fluid builds at the incision, it may clear up on its own or need to be drained off with a needle. Expanders are not recommended for women who are obese, smoke, or have hypertension, diabetes, an infection anywhere in the body, or other health issues. Additional surgery to replace the expander may be required if:

- The expander deflates or leaks.

- A post-operative infection develops.

- Severe capsular contracture of the expander develops.

- The pocket is too large and displaces the expander, making it difficult or impossible to locate the filler port.

Chapter 11

Tummy Tuck Flaps

*Keep a green tree in your heart,
and a singing bird will come.*

– Chinese proverb

When surgeons first began reconstructing breasts, their goal was simply to give women something better than a prosthesis to fill a bra. *Autologous* reconstruction—using a patient's own tissue—creates entirely new possibilities. When skin-sparing mastectomy and tissue flap reconstruction are performed together, surgeons can create natural-looking breasts with minimal scarring. Even women who don't have enough chest muscle to support an implant, or those who had radical mastectomies decades ago, can now have new breasts.

Tissue for breast reconstruction can be borrowed from several donor sites. This chapter describes flap reconstruction using abdominal tissue. These "tummy tuck" methods are two-for-one procedures: the

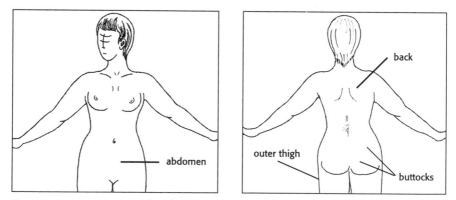

Breasts can be recreated with tissue borrowed from other areas of the body.

same tissue normally removed and discarded after a tummy tuck is used to create the breast. The patient comes out of reconstructive surgery with a new breast *and* a flatter stomach. Before discussing specific abdominal procedures, an overview of tissue flap reconstruction is in order.

Tissue Flap Basics

A breast of your own warm tissue looks and moves like the real thing. When touched, it feels like a breast. Although tissue flaps can't completely restore sensation to the breast—not yet, anyway—women with this type of reconstruction often have more feeling in their new breasts than those with implants.

Autologous reconstruction requires specialized surgical skill; not all plastic surgeons perform these procedures. For the patient, the flap process is more intense than implant reconstruction, but is often completed in less time. The breast mound is shaped in the initial surgery and allowed to settle for a few months before the nipple and areola are created. Sometimes a return trip to the operating room is needed to fine-tune the new breast: remove some fat, revise a scar, or reshape tissue. These revision surgeries are usually minor procedures performed when the nipple is created.

Timeline: Tissue Flap Reconstruction (3-4 months)

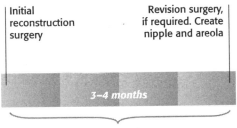

Initial reconstruction surgery

Revision surgery, if required. Create nipple and areola

3–4 months

breast settles

Once shaped into a breast, the new flap must have a healthy blood supply to thrive. That means either leaving the flap attached to its original blood supply at the donor site, or detaching the flap completely and transplanting it in the chest. There are three ways to do this, each requiring a more advanced surgical technique.

Pedicled or *attached flaps* use skin, fat, and muscle from the back or abdomen. The flap is slid under the skin to the mastectomy site and shaped into a breast, but remains attached by a strip of muscle to its original blood supply at the donor site. The biggest drawback of an attached flap is that it sacrifices a perfectly healthy muscle. The muscle itself isn't needed for reconstruction—it's harvested only for the blood vessels it contains, which provide blood flow to the new breast.

Free flaps use only a small portion of muscle at the donor site, so recovery is shorter and less painful than an attached flap. The entire flap, along with its blood supply, is completely removed from the donor site and transplanted to the chest. Free flaps require a skilled *microsurgeon*, a specially trained surgeon who uses a surgical microscope to reconnect the tiny, delicate blood vessels in the flap to blood vessels in the chest or armpit.

Perforator flaps are the gold standard of tissue transfers. They use skin and fat without sacrificing any muscle. The perforators, or arteries feeding the flap, are carefully dissected from the muscle and reconnected to blood vessels in the chest. Few surgeons are qualified to perform this complex operation.

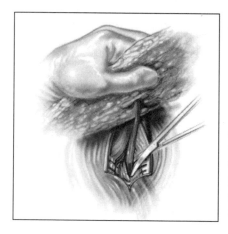

In perforator flap reconstruction, the microsurgeon lifts the flap and carefully extracts tiny blood vessels from the muscle. The flap is transferred to the mastectomy site, where the blood vessels are reconnected to the veins in the chest.

Knowing the possibilities and drawbacks of these three procedures gives you options. You don't have to settle for what any one surgeon can offer you. If you so choose, you can find a surgeon who provides the technique you prefer. When interviewing plastic surgeons, ask which procedures they do, how many they've done, what type of complications they've encountered, and how many patients have had problems.

Borrowing from the abdomen. Abdominal tissue has skin tone and texture similar to breast tissue, so it creates a breast with a natural feel and look. Abdominal flaps can be performed in different ways; the process is easier to grasp if you first understand what's beneath the abdominal skin. Below the tissue and fat are the *rectus abdominis* muscles. You have two: one on the left and one on the right, both extending from below the ribcage to the pubic bone. These are the "six-pack" muscles coveted by bodybuilders. The muscles have two main sources of blood: the *superior* blood vessels at the top of the muscle and the *deep inferior* vessels at the bottom of the muscle.

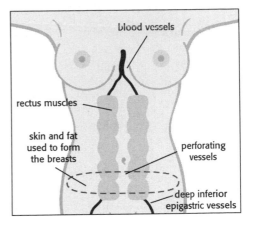

An abdominal flap uses skin, fat, blood vessels, and sometimes muscle to recreate a breast.

The Attached TRAM Flap

Introduced in the 1980s, the *transverse rectus abdominis myocutaneous (TRAM)* flap was the first abdominal transfer technique developed for breast reconstruction. Although it's more complex than implant reconstruction, the attached TRAM is less involved than free or perforator flaps, because it doesn't require microsurgical skill. While it's no longer the most advanced flap reconstruction, TRAM surgery is still the most common, primarily because it's the flap technique most surgeons perform.

How it's done. TRAM surgery begins with a hip-to-hip incision between the navel and pubic bone. A flap of skin, fat, and most of the underlying muscle is cut away and lifted up from the abdomen. A strip of muscle remains, acting as an umbilical cord and supplying blood between the flap and the abdomen. Most of one rectus abdominis muscle is used for unilateral reconstruction. A larger flap and both muscles are used in bilateral reconstruction or to recreate a very large breast.

The flap is turned upward and tunneled under the skin to the mastectomy site. The upper part of the flap is sewn into position to provide fullness at the top of the new breast. The lower flap is folded under, shaped to match the size and shape of the opposite breast, and sutured in place. At this point,

Unilateral Attached TRAM		
Surgery		3–6 hours
Hospital stay immediate delayed		4–8 days
Back to daily activities		4–8 weeks
Back to sports and strenuous activities		3–6 months

many surgeons bring their patients to a sitting position to adjust the symmetry between the breasts. To finish the operation, the abdominal muscle edges are sewn together. The upper and lower portions of the abdominal incision are pulled together and sutured closed.

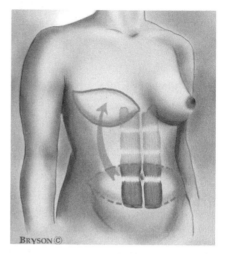

In an attached TRAM procedure, a flap of skin, fat, and most of the rectus abdominus muscle (top) is tunneled under the skin to the chest. When delayed reconstruction is performed, re-excising the mastectomy scar creates an elliptical opening through which the flap is pulled and shaped into a breast (bottom left). The remaining scar encircles the new breast (bottom right). BRYSON ©

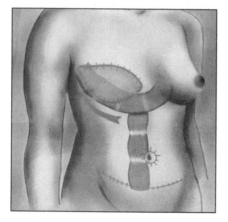

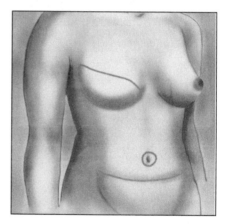

To improve blood flow, some surgeons perform a *delay* procedure (not to be confused with delayed reconstruction) a week or two before the flap operation. The blood vessels in the lower abdomen are divided to encourage the blood vessels in the upper abdomen—the ones that will supply the flap with blood—to grow. This minor procedure involves two short incisions made along the same lines as the flap surgery, so you don't get any additional scars.

TRAM surgery can only be done once. If a second reconstruction is required at a later time, an implant or tissue from a different donor site must be used. If you don't have enough abdominal tissue for bilateral reconstruction, a different donor site can be used to create the second breast.

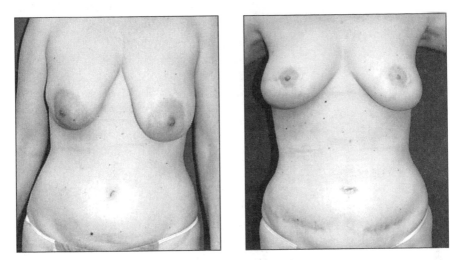

A patient before an immediate bilateral TRAM reconstruction (top left) and after (top right). Another patient before her delayed TRAM reconstruction (bottom left) and after (bottom right). Opening the mastectomy scar to accommodate the flap creates an elliptical scar on the new breast. Her nipple and areola will be added in a later procedure.

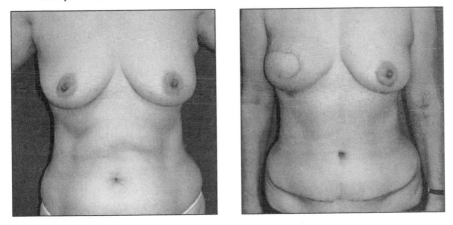

Recovery. TRAM surgery is serious business. Recovery can be tough and very uncomfortable, particularly after an attached TRAM procedure. You'll feel like a tractor rolled over you. You're recovering from not one, but two significant operations and the loss of one or both major abdominal muscles. For the first couple of weeks, your

When I woke up from my TRAM operation, I felt as though I had been hit by a bus. The first week or so, I thought I'd made a terrible mistake. It did get better each day, but the first week was awful. I couldn't stand or sit up straight for almost three weeks. – Teri

Honestly, my TRAM hurt like hell. I spent a lot of the day crying and just stayed on medication until I got better. Now I'm just as excited about my flat stomach as I am my new breast. For the first time in my life, I'm a babe! I'm wearing clothes I never would have worn before my surgery. – Monique

movement will be limited. You'll be given pain medication around the clock, and you'll have surgical drains at the mastectomy and donor sites.

Women with strong abdominal muscles and good overall health fare better than those who are overweight or don't exercise. Doing sit-ups and other abdominal exercises regularly four to six weeks before your surgery will strengthen your muscles and increase blood flow.

It's amazing how many movements involve the abdominal muscles. That's something you'll discover after your TRAM operation. Sitting, standing, bending over, getting out of bed, and other movements we take for granted will be difficult until your incision begins to heal. You'll be encouraged to get up and walk a little the first day or two after surgery. It won't be easy, but the nurse will help you. You probably won't be able to stand straight for a couple of weeks. Pain medication will help, but you'll have limited range of motion in your arms and chest, and your abdomen will be very tight and sore.

You'll feel a pulling sensation in your abdomen for three to six months or more. The area around your incision may remain numb for several months until the nerves regenerate. You'll have to sleep on your back for several weeks until your abdomen and chest heal. You may have to give yourself a boost to get out of bed or up from a chair during this time. If you've had bilateral TRAM reconstruction, you may need help getting in and out of bed for a couple of weeks.

Smaller meals will feel better with your newly tightened abdomen. Caffeine can reduce the blood supply to the flap—it's a good idea to avoid chocolate, coffee, tea, or any other products with caffeine for a few weeks. You shouldn't wear a bra, drive, engage in sex, or lift more than five pounds for at least three weeks or until cleared by your doctor.

You can gradually begin more vigorous movement and should be back to most routine activities within two months. You many feel tired for several more weeks, but will gradually improve. It will take three to six months to return to golf, tennis, lifting weights, or other strenuous activities.

For the first two or three months after your surgery, your reconstructed breast will be swollen and look fuller than its final size. It will be larger than your other breast. As the swelling subsides and the muscle thins from lack of exercise, your new breast will take on its final shape.

Scarring. No matter what type flap is used, abdominal reconstruction leaves a very prominent scar at the panty line. It will be covered by most bathing suits, but will show in a bikini. Talk to your surgeon before your operation about the exact placement of your scar. You'll also have a thin scar around your navel, as described later in this chapter.

My cousin had a TRAM flap the year before I did. I was about 20 pounds overweight, but she was in good shape. Her first seven or eight days were painful, and then she made steady improvement. I had quite a bit of pain for more than three weeks.
– Carrie

Remember, reconstruction is performed through the mastectomy incision or scar. If you have a skin-sparing mastectomy with immediate TRAM, you'll have a thin scar around the areola, which will be mostly covered by your new areola. You may also have a short scar to either side of the areola. A delayed reconstruction scar is much larger, as described in Chapter 4. Unlike delayed implant reconstruction, which produces a straight scar line across the new breast, delayed tissue flap reconstruction results in an elliptical scar around the breast. The scars on your abdomen and breast are permanent, but will fade in time.

Potential Problems. Most women have no long-term effects from an attached TRAM, other than an inability to do sit-ups. Complications can occur, however, including the following.

- Abdominal weakness. An attached TRAM reconstruction can cause long-term abdominal weakness, which may limit routine activities, particularly for someone who is athletic. Some women never fully regain their previous abdominal strength. Others experience back weakness or feel unbalanced and need physical therapy to deal with the muscle loss.

- Slow healing. Incisions are sometimes slow to heal and may prolong your recovery period.

- Hernia. Removing much of the rectus abdominis muscle weakens the abdominal wall. This can result in hernia, a bulge under the skin caused when the intestines poke through the weakened muscle. Hernia used to be the most common problem after an attached TRAM, particularly with bilateral reconstruction. Most surgeons now reinforce the abdomen with surgical mesh—hernias occur in less than five percent of TRAM patients. If the problem does occur, it can be quite painful and requires surgery to repair the muscle.

Several months after my TRAM, I developed what I called my third boob. It was this A-cup size lump sticking out above my waistline. My doctor said it was the result of tunneling the flap up under the skin. It did finally shrink, but it took almost a year.
– B.J.

- Lumps and bulges. A lump is the last thing a cancer patient wants to find in her new breast, but non-cancerous lumps commonly occur after attached TRAM surgery. Sliding the flap under the skin can disturb the tissue between abdomen and chest, causing bulges under the skin, particularly when the patient is thin. A glob of fat may poke up under the skin or the flap edge becomes hard. Your surgeon may use a needle to aspirate the lump to determine the cause. If the lump doesn't soften on its own in a few months, it is usually removed surgically or with liposuction.

- Necrosis. Infrequently, a portion of the flap doesn't get enough blood. If this happens, part of your new breast may feel hard or thick. You may simply leave it alone. If it bothers you, your surgeon can remove the dead tissue in a minor office operation. Rarely, the entire flap dies and requires an entirely new reconstruction.

- Infection. Infection is unusual, but is possible with any surgery. It's more likely to occur in women who smoke, are obese, have diabetes or have had radiation or chemotherapy. Infections are treated with antibiotics.

- Seroma and Hematoma. If a seroma or a hematoma forms, it may disappear on its own or can be drained with a needle.

The Free TRAM

Microsurgeons can now harvest abdominal flaps without sacrificing the entire muscle. In free TRAM reconstruction, the entire flap and its blood supply are lifted clear of the abdomen and transplanted to the mastectomy site. Only a small portion of the muscle used. The artery and veins feeding the flap are reconnected to the blood supply in the underarm. While an attached TRAM uses vessels from the upper abdomen, a free TRAM uses the lower or *superior* vessels. This provides a more robust blood flow to the new breast.

Recovery. Recovery from a free TRAM isn't as intensely painful as an attached TRAM, but it can still be uncomfortable, particularly during the first week. Because microsurgery is involved, a free TRAM is a longer and more complex operation than an attached TRAM procedure.

Unilateral Free TRAM	
Surgery	6-8 hours
Hospital stay immediate or delayed	4-7 days
Back to daily activities	4-6 weeks
Back to sports and strenuous activities	3-6 months

Potential problems. Preserving most of the muscle retains abdominal function and strength. There's no need for surgical mesh and little risk of hernia. The flap is transplanted to the mastectomy site, so under-the-skin bulges aren't a problem.

Problems occur infrequently. Occasionally, inadequate circulation to the flap can delay healing. The incision takes longer to heal and may begin weeping, or leaking fluid or blood. Because the blood supply must be cut and reconnected at the mastectomy site, initial blood supply to the flap is not as reliable as an attached TRAM procedure. Blockage of the blood vessels feeding the new breast is a more serious, but less common problem. If this occurs, the flap may die and the entire reconstruction must be repeated using a different technique. This happens infrequently. The risk of flap loss is less than three percent.

The DIEP Flap

Why sacrifice a perfectly good muscle if you don't have to? That's the philosophy behind the *Deep Inferior Epigastric Perforator (DIEP)* flap. Developed in Germany in the early 1990s, DIEP reconstruction is the most advanced flap procedure. The DIEP or perforator flap uses the same amount of tissue and fat as the attached and free TRAM flaps, but preserves all the muscle. The microsurgeon extracts the tiny arteries from the muscle and reconnects them to the blood supply in the chest.

Unilateral DIEP Flap	
Surgery	6-8 hours
Hospital stay immediate or delayed	3-5 days
Back to daily activities	4-5 weeks
Back to sports and strenuous activities	3-4 months

DIEP surgery is far more complex, and therefore longer, than the attached and free TRAM methods. Because the underlying muscle is undisturbed, recovery is somewhat shorter and less painful. Risk of hernia is less than one percent. Abdominal weakness and complication is also greatly reduced compared to TRAM procedures. Women who can't have TRAM reconstruction because of previous abdominal surgery, excessive weight, or other circulatory problems may be candidates for a DIEP procedure.

I play a lot of tennis, so I was in pretty good shape before my surgery. I wanted to get back on the court as soon as possible, so I had a DIEP operation. I was out of it for several days, but I recovered well and was back to most of my routine in about a month. – Casey

Improved sensation. One very exciting advantage of a DIEP reconstruction is the potential for improved sensation in the new breast. Women with flap reconstruction often regain more rudimentary sensations of pressure, warmth, and coldness than women with implants. This is due to nerves in the flap spontaneously connecting with nerves in the chest. It appears more sensation is regained if the surgeon reconnects the flap's *intercostal* nerve to a cut nerve at the mastectomy site. It's a slow process. It may take a year or more for the nerves to regenerate. Limited sensation increases after two or three years beyond reconstruction.

Nerve restoration is the next frontier in reconstruction. If surgeons can restore sensation, reconstruction will almost completely reestablish a woman's breast after mastectomy. Undoubtedly, this will require even greater, more specialized surgical skill. Ongoing studies at Johns Hopkins University are exploring the possibilities.

Finding a DIEP surgeon. DIEP is superior to TRAM, but it takes a lot more training and experience. Only a few U.S. surgeons are skilled at this technique, but it is catching on. Many women consider it worth while to have one of these surgeons perform their reconstruction, even if it means traveling out of state or across the country. If you'd like to consider the DIEP method, here are some of the surgeons who are qualified to perform the procedure:

1. **San Diego**
   Dr. Gilbert Lee
   (858-720-1440 or www.changesplasticsurgery.com)

2. **Dallas**
   Dr. Frederick Duffy
   (972-566-3939 or www.dallasdiep.com)

3. New Orleans
Dr. Robert Allen
(504-894-2900 or www.diepflap.com)

Dr. Allen has been performing DIEP procedures since 1992 and is widely credited as the American authority on DIEP reconstruction.

4. Miami Beach
Dr. Gary Rosenbaum
(305-538-7726 or www.drgaryrosenbaum.com)

5. Baltimore
Dr. Bernard Chang
(410-332-9700 or www.mdmercy.com/PlasticSurgery)

6. Baltimore
Dr. Maurice Nahabedian
(410-955-8964 or www.hopkinsmedicine.org/breastcenter/)

7. Great Neck
Dr. Alex Keller
(516-482-1100 or www.breastflap.com)

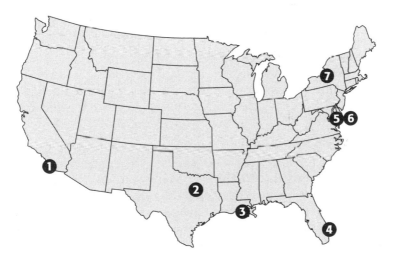

Paying for DIEP reconstruction. If your health plan allows you to choose any doctor, you may have no problem with payment for DIEP reconstruction. A managed care plan is more likely to require that you use an in-network surgeon. It's unlikely any of the contracted surgeons are qualified to perform DIEP flaps, however, so your insurer may approve going out of network for your operation. Another argument in favor of DIEP is the shorter hospital stay and fewer post-operative complications compared to other abdominal flap operations. Contact your health care administrator regarding payment. You may have to be persistent. Your insurance company may not even be aware of the DIEP procedure. The surgeon's office staff can help you deal with insurance issues, and if you travel for your surgery, they can direct you to nearby hotels.

Building a New Belly Button

If you've always wished your innie was an outie, or vice versa, you'll get your wish as a by-product of your reconstruction. Removing tissue from the abdomen pulls the navel off-center. This is a common by-product of tummy tucks as well as TRAM and DIEP surgeries. Sometimes the belly button can be repositioned, but surgeons usually create a new one.

Shaping a new navel takes about 30 minutes. It can be done during the initial reconstruction, later when the nipple and areola are created, or as a separate outpatient mini-surgery. The surgeon first marks the new center of the stomach. Using very small incisions, he removes the fat just beneath the skin. This forms an indentation when the incisions are closed.

Is a TRAM or DIEP Right for You?

Abdominal flap reconstruction is major surgery. You must be well enough to withstand the long operation and the recovery. If you've had a gall bladder operation, liposuction, or other abdominal surgery that cut through the upper rectus abdominis muscle, a free TRAM or DIEP may be a better option than an attached TRAM. A previous Caesarean section, however, doesn't necessarily preclude you from having reconstruction with an abdominal flap. If you're thin, you may not have enough tummy flab for a flap. If you are obese, suffer from hypertension or chronic diabetes, or have had previous radiation to the abdomen, your surgeon will assess your condition and advise whether you can have reconstruction at all. In all cases, the decision to proceed with abdominal surgery is assessed on an individual basis.

Smoking is another problem altogether. It compromises any surgery, particularly one so dependent on a healthy blood supply. Smokers have increased risk of blood clotting. They also experience higher rates of post-surgical infection and other complications. A study at M.D. Anderson Cancer Center assessed the effects of smoking in 718 women with free TRAM reconstruction. Smokers experienced higher rates of flap necrosis and hernia than non-smokers and ex-smokers. Smoking-related problems were significantly reduced when women stopped smoking at least four weeks before surgery.

How TRAM affects future pregnancies. If pregnancy is a future possibility, it's better to have a free TRAM, a DIEP flap, or reconstruction with tissue from a different donor site. A bilateral attached TRAM is not advised, because the remaining muscle may not be strong enough to support the baby to term. Talk with your gynecologist and surgeon before you decide on your method of reconstruction.

Comparing Abdominal Flaps and Implants

Implants or abdominal flaps? Which reconstructive procedure best fits your needs? If you're thinking about reconstruction, you'll want to consider the advantages and disadvantages of both procedures. Studies at the University of Michigan surveyed women to determine their satisfaction with reconstruction one year after surgery. (The study did not include women with DIEP reconstruction.)

Michigan Breast Reconstruction Outcome Study (MBROS)	TRAM	IMPLANTS
Overall satisfied with reconstruction	78%	61%
Very satisfied with reconstruction	75%	40%

Note: One year after surgery, none of the women had problems performing routine activities, but women with implant reconstruction were more able to do sit-ups than those with attached or free TRAM reconstruction.

Advantages of TRAM or DIEP reconstruction

- Results in a flatter stomach.

- Easier to create symmetry without altering the opposite breast.

- Provides an alternative for women who don't want synthetic materials in their bodies.

- The new breast gains and loses weight with the rest of your body. and is more likely to retain symmetry with your opposite breast over time.

- Shorter reconstructive process. A tissue transfer patient wakes up with a fully developed breast in place. She needs only the nipple procedure, and possibly a minor touch-up, to finish her breast. A woman with expanders needs several more weeks to grow her breast mound. She must have additional surgery to exchange the expander for an implant before her nipple is constructed.

- Offers a better chance of increased sensation in the new breast.

- Fewer long-term complications. Flaps don't leak or rupture, and only rarely must be replaced.

- Radiation is less likely to compromise the quality of the reconstructed breast.

Disadvantages of TRAM or DIEP reconstruction

- Scars an otherwise healthy part of the body.

- Exposes the patient to anesthesia for a longer time.

- Recovery is more uncomfortable.

- Attached TRAM may permanently decrease abdominal strength.

- More likely to require additional surgery to adjust the shape or size of the breast.

- More difficult to find qualified surgeons, particularly for DIEP reconstruction.

Chapter 12

Other Flap Methods

**Shoot for the moon. Even if you miss,
you'll land among the stars.**
– Les Brown

If you're not eligible for a TRAM or DIEP procedure, or you don't want to be left with a long scar across your abdomen, flaps can be taken from the back, buttocks, or thighs. Although these procedures are used less often than implants or abdominal flaps, they produce very good reconstructive results.

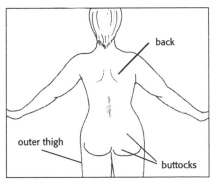

Flap reconstruction can be accomplished with tissue from the back, buttocks, or outer thigh.

The Back Flap

The *latissimus dorsi* or back flap reconstruction uses the long, flat muscle below the shoulder. Unlike an abdominal flap, the tissue and skin from the back have a somewhat different texture and skin tone than a natural breast; the new breast may look and feel slightly different.

This technique was originally developed for women who had radical mastectomies. The latissimus dorsi muscle replaced the missing

As an aerobics instructor, I didn't want to risk reduced abdominal strength, even though my doctor said I'd be okay after TRAM reconstruction. I read about the back flap in a magazine. It took a while to find a surgeon who was qualified to do it, but I'm glad I did. – DeeDee

chest muscle and the flap of skin and fat provided enough healthy tissue to cover an implant. Back flap reconstruction became less popular once TRAM techniques were developed. It's an alternative for women without enough abdominal fat to create a breast, or those who can't have TRAM or DIEP surgery due to health conditions, previous abdominal surgery, or radiation to the abdomen.

Reconstruction with a back flap is relatively easy surgery with a reliable blood supply, good results, and few problems. If the reconstructed breast is small, a back flap may be sufficient. Most often, however, an implant is also needed. It gives the new breast volume while the flap provides the muscle to cover it. This is not a good reconstructive method for women with back or shoulder problems, or who have had surgery in the armpit, which can potentially disrupt blood flow to the flap.

How it's done. A back flap operation begins with the patient on her side. The surgeon makes a 4-to-6 inch incision below the shoulder blade. This is an attached flap procedure: the skin, fat, and part of the muscle are tunneled under the skin, across the armpit, and to the mastectomy site. The flap remains connected to its blood supply in the back.

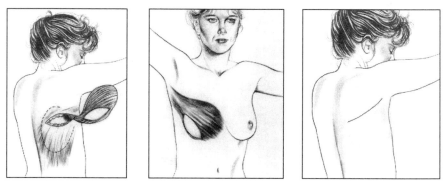

The back flap is tunneled under the skin to the mastectomy site (left). An implant is often used to add volume to the breast (center). The flap leaves a scar beneath the shoulder blade (right).

If you're considering latissimus dorsi reconstruction, it's worth finding an *endoscopic* surgeon. Your scar will be much smaller and your recovery less painful than with a traditional back flap. The reconstruction is done entirely through the mastectomy incision or a small incision under the arm. Using a special surgical tool, the surgeon creates the flap and moves it in place.

Extended latissimus dorsi reconstruction is a free flap variation on the technique. A larger flap of skin and fat is removed and transplanted at the chest, so the breast is reconstructed without an implant. This does result in a considerably longer scar down the back that may show in swimsuits, tank tops, and sundresses.

The Back Flap	
Surgery	3-6 hours
Hospital stay immediate or delayed	4-8 days
Back to daily activities	4-8 weeks
Back to sports and strenuous activities	3-6 months

Recovery. Recovery is not as long or as painful as a TRAM operation. The donor site tends to collect more fluid after surgery than other methods of reconstruction. Surgical drains remain at the new breast and in the back for two to three weeks. The back will be numb for a few months until the nerves grow back. The upper back may be sore for five or six weeks, but any discomfort is usually controlled with over-the-counter pain medications. You may also experience soreness under your arm from tunneling the flap around to the chest.

Potential problems. Back flap reconstruction is generally free of problems. Because it's an attached flap, the blood supply is very reliable: less than two percent of patients experience necrosis. The most common problem is seroma in women who are obese or over age 65.

Bulges sometimes occur under the arm from tunneling the flap to the chest. As the muscle atrophies over time, the bulge shrinks, but may never disappear completely. Infections are uncommon, but are generally treated successfully with antibiotics if they do occur. If an implant is used, the patient is subject to the inherent problems discussed in Chapter 9.

Removing the lat muscle causes some asymmetry in the back. Generally, this doesn't cause significant weakness or interfere with routine activities, but some women notice reduced performance when

I'm the world's biggest chicken when it comes to pain. I asked my doctor what method of reconstruction was the least painful. He recommended using the muscle in my back and a small implant. My recovery wasn't bad and my new breast is fine.
– Marta

swimming, golfing, climbing, playing tennis, or other activities that depend heavily on shoulder or back strength.

Advantages of the back flap

- Provides a reliable method of reconstruction.

- The flap is easily shaped into a breast.

- Doesn't restrict or weaken normal movement after recovery.

- Recovery is shorter and less painful than abdominal flaps.

Disadvantages of the back flap

- Most women will also need an implant.

- Leaves a long scar down the back (unless endoscopic surgery is performed).

- Usually provides only enough tissue to create an A or B cup breast.

- The patient must be turned from her side to her back during surgery.

- The new breast has a different skin tone and texture than the opposite breast.

Gluteal Flaps

Posterior, derriere, fanny, rump, tush, gluteus maximus. Popular jargon aside, a well-padded bottom can be a prime source of soft, natural tissue for reconstruction. Although gluteal flaps are performed less frequently than other reconstructive procedures, they produce very good results for women who don't have enough tissue in the back or abdomen. Even slender women usually have enough buttock tissue to create a moderately sized breast. Like the TRAM procedure, this free flap comes with a bonus of its own: a higher, firmer buttock.

Gluteal flaps can be taken from the upper or lower buttock, depending where the most fatty tissue and best blood supply are located. The *superior gluteal* flap uses skin and tissue from the upper buttock. It's more difficult to harvest. The incision is made just below the bikini line, so the scar is usually hidden under swimsuits.

The *inferior gluteal* flap uses tissue from the lower buttock and a small portion of the *gluteus maximus* muscle. The incision is made in the buttock crease. This is a very difficult and demanding operation—the surgeon must be very careful not to nick or cut the sciatic or gluteal motor nerves. The tissue is more difficult to shape than a soft abdominal flap, but produces a very natural breast. If your breast is reconstructed with this method, your flap scar will be hidden in the crease, but you'll feel it for several months to a year every time you sit down.

The *superior gluteal artery perforator* or *S-GAP* flap is similar to the DIEP technique. A flap of tissue with its blood supply is completely removed from the buttocks and reattached in the chest. No muscle is removed.

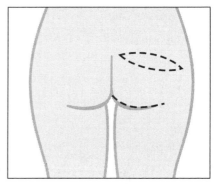

Gluteal flaps can be taken from the upper or lower buttock.

Because gluteal flap reconstructions are complex long procedures, they are almost never done at the same time as mastectomy. Two surgeons perform the operation. While one is harvesting the flap, the other is preparing the mastectomy site. Like the back flap, the patient starts the operation on her side, and then is turned on her back to position the flap. Bilateral reconstruction is always done in two stages; only one gluteal flap can be harvested at a time.

Recovery. After surgery, you'll feel a dull ache in the area around the incision, but a gluteal flap isn't as painful as TRAM surgery. You'll be tender for several days, but will be mobile by the second or third day. You should be walking comfortably after the first week and ready to go home from the hospital.

During gluteal surgery, the nerve in the back of the leg is cut where it enters the buttock. The back of the thigh will be numb until this nerve grows back. It may take several weeks or up to six months or a year until you regain feeling.

You'll have a drain in your chest, which will be removed in a few days. An additional drain at the buttock may remain in place for

The day I came home from the hospital, my 7-year old ran next door to tell the neighbors that Mommy's new boob came from her bottom. – Carmel

The best thing about the gluteal scar is that I don't have to see it every time I look in the mirror. – Sondra

another week or two. An inflatable donut pillow—the kind used by hemorrhoid sufferers—will make sitting more comfortable. You'll need to sleep on the opposite side until your incision heals.

Borrowing tissue from this large muscle group doesn't permanently impair strength or functional movement, but it does flatten the buttock somewhat. Symmetry can be restored by removing an equal amount of tissue from the other buttock with surgery or liposuction.

Advantages of the gluteal flap

- Donor scar is hidden by underwear.

- No loss of muscle function or strength.

- Most women have enough buttock tissue to create a breast.

- Provides an alternative for women who can't have abdominal or back flaps.

Disadvantages of the gluteal flap

- Operation is long and complex.

- Patient must be turned during procedure.

- Unilateral flap causes buttock asymmetry.

- Bilateral reconstruction must be done in two phases.

- Potential for injury to gluteal or sciatic nerves.

- Sitting is uncomfortable for several months until the scar heals.

The Thigh Flap

The *lateral transverse thigh* flap, also called the Reubens flap, uses tissue from the upper or outer thigh. This procedure is only performed as a last resort for women who don't have enough tissue anywhere else. While it's nice to be rid of saddlebags, this free flap operation leaves a long, obvious scar on the leg. A unilateral flap causes very visible asymmetry with the opposite leg. Recovery and potential problems are similar to those of a free TRAM. Because seroma is a common problem, surgical drains may be required for a longer time than other flap procedures.

Chapter 13

Altering the Opposite Breast

*Being happy doesn't mean everything's perfect;
it just means you've decided to see beyond the
imperfections.*

– Unknown

Reconstruction will give you a nicely shaped new breast, but will it match the other side? When a surgeon recreates both breasts, he can ensure they're of similar size and shape. Unilateral reconstruction presents a different problem: how to achieve balance between the reconstructed breast and your natural breast?

Most women will need an operation on their opposite breast to achieve the best possible symmetry. Your reconstructed breast won't be an exact match—even natural breasts are never identical. Often, however, reconstructing one breast and altering the other produces a very good match. It's possible to complete reconstruction with bigger, smaller, higher, or firmer breasts than before your mastectomy. This opportunity for a breast makeover is something many women may have long considered but never pursued.

If you would rather not scar a perfectly healthy breast, choose a reconstructive technique that can best match it. If your natural breasts are small and firm, for example, implant reconstruction is a good choice. Tissue flap reconstruction can better match a breast that is flat, very small, very large, or quite droopy.

Three surgical procedures are used to modify the opposite breast:

Augmentation uses an implant to increase the size of your breast.

Reduction makes your breast smaller by removing skin and tissue.

Lift creates a higher breast by removing skin. This procedure is often combined with augmentation to make a fuller, higher breast.

Planning your surgery. If you decide to have a little work done on your natural breast, review your surgeon's before-and-after photos of reconstruction patients who have had the same surgery. Notice how closely (or not) their reconstructed and modified breasts match. Ask your surgeon to explain the best and worst results you can expect and where your scars will be.

Your reconstructed breast mound is given time to assume its final shape before any changes are made to your opposite breast. This may take two to four months. You'll be somewhat lopsided during this period until your healthy breast is altered.

Check with your health provider to determine conditions of payment. If the company pays for your reconstruction, it must also pay for modifications to your other breast to achieve symmetry. If it doesn't cover reconstruction, it will probably not pay for cosmetic procedures to your opposite breast. Some insurers require changes be made at the same time as the reconstruction.

About cosmetic breast procedures. Although the procedures described in this chapter aren't as lengthy or as complex as reconstruction, you'll feel the after effects. Initially, you'll need pain medication to control your discomfort. You'll be out of bed within a day or two, but may feel tired and won't feel like doing much for five to seven days. Take advantage of the time to rest, relax and allow yourself to heal.

Most women have no complications after surgery, but there's always the risk of excessive bleeding or a negative reaction to anesthesia. The potential for infection will be limited by antibiotics given before and after surgery. Call your doctor immediately if you have bleeding through your bandages, persistent pain, or other unusual symptoms.

Follow your surgeon's pre-operative and post-operative instructions. He'll suggest exercises to restore the range of motion in your arm and chest, and will tell you when you can return to work and resume normal activities. Stick to sponge baths until your stitches are removed.

Be careful not to lift, pull, or push until he says it's okay to do so. Don't pick up your children or the laundry. Have someone help you around the house for the first 48 hours after surgery. Until your incision heals, avoid any activities that can raise your blood pressure, including sexual activity—excess blood at the incision can cause swelling and hinder healing.

Don't be surprised if your altered breast is too high, too low, too small, too big, or misshapen after surgery. This is to be expected until the bruising and swelling disappear and your breast takes on its final look. If needed, minor revision surgery to fine-tune the breast size, shape, or position can be done when your nipple is created.

Your scars may remain red and lumpy for several months, but in time will fade to thinner, white lines that will be covered by most bras, lingerie, and bathing suits. Some women's breast scars are barely visible. Others have very conspicuous scars, particularly after breast reduction. Ask your surgeon what you should expect.

Reducing or lifting the breast often involve recentering the nipple and areola. This may cause a permanent loss of some or all sensation in that area.

Breast Augmentation

Augmentation mammoplasty or breast enlargement increases your breast by a full cup size or more. Adding an implant will make your breast fuller and firmer but not necessarily higher.

How it's done. Breast augmentation is a relatively easy operation. It can be done under general or local anesthetic. Most augmentation is performed through a 1-to-3 inch incision in the crease under the breast. A longer incision is required to accommodate textured or silicone implants. Less frequently, the incision is made in the armpit. This axillary cut makes for a more difficult surgery and leaves a permanent scar which will show when you raise your arm. Some surgeons use a *periareolar* cut around the areola.

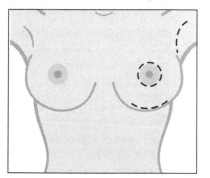

Augmentation is performed through an incision around the areola, in the underarm, or in the crease under the breast.

Augmentation surgery is similar to the pocket procedure used for implant reconstruction. An implant is placed into a pocket created behind the chest muscle. This creates a fuller shape by pushing the breast tissue forward. Placing the implant behind the muscle serves two purposes: it better matches the position of the reconstructed implanted breast and it reduces the risk of capsular contracture. There is no need for expansion.

Once the implant is in place, the surgical team sits you up to ensure your augmented breast is positioned to match your reconstructed breast. The surgeon closes the incision with small, fine stitches and binds the breast with gauze dressing, a surgical compression bandage, or a surgical bra.

Recovery. After surgery, your chest will feel heavy for several days, as if a gorilla is sitting there. Your breast may be bruised, swollen, and sore for two to four weeks. Cold compresses or ice packs will help reduce the swelling. Your breast may be too high and excessively firm, but it will drop and soften over the next few weeks as your skin and muscle stretch to accommodate the implant.

You may feel tingling, burning sensations, or sharp pains for a few weeks. Your nipples may be very sensitive; even rubbing against clothing may make them itch or ache. Covering your nipple with a small round Band-Aid until the sensitivity disappears may help.

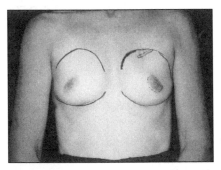

Markings outline the pocket area (top) before mastectomy and implant reconstruction of the left breast and augmentation of the right breast (bottom left). After nipple reconstruction, the breasts are closely matched (bottom right). Augmentation through an underarm incision leaves the healthy breast unscarred. The reconstructed breast shows the biopsy scar and barely-visible scars around the areola.

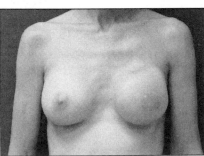

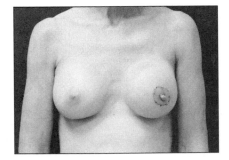

Most women can shower and return to restricted activities and work without heavy lifting within a week. Some women require a few more days to recover. In three to four weeks you should regain normal range of motion and resume routine activities. After six to eight weeks, the swelling subsides and you'll be able to see the changes in your breast.

Potential complications. Less than two percent of women who have augmentation lose some or all feeling in their nipple and areola, and sometimes throughout the breast. If this occurs, it cannot be resolved.

Women who nurse their babies within the year prior to augmentation may produce milk for several days after their operation. Your surgeon can control this with prescribed medication. If you augment your breast with a silicone implant and plan to breastfeed in the future, you may be interested in a 1998 study at Women's College Health Sciences Center. It found the level of silicone in breast milk wasn't significantly different in women who had silicone implants than those who didn't.

All implants, whether used for reconstruction or augmentation, are subject to the potential problems described in Chapter 9.

Breast Augmentation	
Surgery	1-2 hours
Hospital stay	None
Back to daily activities	I week
Back to sports and strenuous activities	3-4 weeks

When an implant is placed behind the muscle, it doesn't interfere with future breast examinations or mammograms. You should have a baseline mammogram before your breast is augmented and have all future mammograms of that breast evaluated by specially trained health care professionals.

Breast Reduction

Reduction mammoplasty or breast reduction greatly improves the shape and size of large, saggy breasts. If you're bothered by rashes, breathing problems, pain, or other complications from breasts that are too big, reduction can boost your self-image and make life a lot more comfortable. After reduction, you'll have a smaller, lighter breast in better proportion to your body. Be sure to communicate clearly with your surgeon about how much tissue should be removed. Bring a photo of how you would like to look, or a bra you would like to fit into. Look at his before-and-after photos of reconstruction patients who have had their opposite breast reduced. Ask your surgeon how and where the incisions will be made.

How it's done. Reduction is a more complex procedure than augmentation. It involves removing excess tissue, fat, and skin, and then sewing the breast back together. It can be done in a number of different ways, depending on your surgeon's preferred technique and how much tissue is to be removed.

Reduction is often performed through an anchor incision—a combination of periareolar and inframammary cuts connected by a vertical incision from the nipple to the crease. The breast is then opened and excess tissue is removed. When only a small amount of tissue is to be removed, the entire reduction can be done through a periareolar incision.

During the operation, the nipple usually remains attached to its nerves and blood vessels on an island of skin. This little island is pulled up and out of the way until the excess tissue is removed. If the breasts are very large, however, it may be necessary to completely remove the nipple and graft it to a higher position. If this occurs, feeling in the nipple may be permanently lost.

Once the excess tissue has been removed, the nipple is recentered. Skin from both sides of the breast is brought down and together, creating a firmer, tighter contour. A surgical drain is placed at the site,

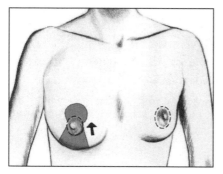

The breast is opened with an anchor incision and excess tissue and fat is removed (top). The nipple and areola are recentered on the reduced breast and the incisions are pulled together (bottom left). The newly reduced breast more closely matches the reconstructed breast (bottom right).

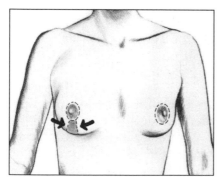

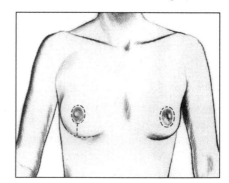

and the newly reduced breast is wrapped in elastic bandages or a surgical compression bra.

Blood transfusions are rarely required, but if your breasts are very large and quite a bit of tissue will be removed, your surgeon may suggest you donate one or two units of blood a few weeks before your surgery, just in case it's needed.

This woman's natural breasts sagged considerably (left). Several months after her right breast was reconstructed with expansion and an implant, her left breast was reduced and lifted (right).

Recovery. Breast reduction is a serious operation; recovery can be very uncomfortable. Most pain occurs in the first three or four days after surgery, particularly if you move excessively, cough, or sneeze. After that, you'll be up and around, but restricted from lifting or exerting too much.

Your bandages will be removed in two to three days. In about two weeks, your stitches will come out and you may return to work. Most women are back to full activities in three to four weeks. Your reduced breast may be especially sensitive and swollen during your first menstrual period after surgery.

You'll need to wear a sports bra around the clock for a few weeks until the swelling subsides. Your nipple and breast may be numb for six to eight weeks or longer. Feeling returns gradually as the swelling subsides. Some women, however, remain numb for a year or more. It may take six months to a year to heal completely.

Breast reduction can leave thick, prominent scars. If you gain weight after your surgery, your reduced breast may regain some or all of its previous size. If your missing breast is reconstructed with a tissue flap, it, too, will reflect future weight gains or losses. Implanted breasts, however, will not.

Potential complications. A small percentage of women who have breast reduction lose some or all feeling in their nipples, and sometimes permanently lose sensation in the breast. In very rare cases, the nipple and areola may die from loss of blood supply. If this occurs, a skin graft is required to rebuild the nipple. Some women experience sharp, shooting pains until their breast heals completely.

Breast Reduction	
Surgery	1-3 hours
Hospital stay	None or overnight
Back to daily Activities	3-4 weeks
Back to sports and strenuous activities	4-6 week

If your nipple is removed during surgery, the milk ducts will be severed and the chance of breast-feeding is reduced. Milk ducts may also be severed when excess tissue is removed. Your ability to breast-feed is more likely to be preserved when the nipple is left attached to the skin and the milk ducts are left intact. If you're concerned about this, discuss the procedure with your surgeon. The BreastFeeding After Reduction (BFAR) website provides information and support to mothers who want to breastfeed after reduction surgery (www.bfar.org).

Breast Lift

All breasts head south over time. As tissue loses elasticity, breasts hang lower on the chest and areolae become larger. This *ptosis,* or sagging, results from age, excess weight, pregnancy, hormones, or genetics. If you want to change the look and position, but not the size, of your breast, a *mastopexy* will raise it higher on your chest.

How it's done. During a mastopexy, a section of skin is removed from the breast and the remaining skin edges are sewn together. Afterwards, you have the same amount of breast tissue held together by less skin, so your breast is higher and tighter. Small saggy breasts can be lifted and augmented. Overly large breasts can be lifted and reduced.

The type of incision depends on the amount of skin to be removed and the technique favored by your surgeon. If your breast is small with minimal sagging, he may remove only a crescent-shaped segment of skin from above your areola. A periareolar or lollipop incision is used to improve a moderately sagging breast. Lifting a heavily sagging breast may require an anchor incision.

Once the incision is made, the predetermined amount of skin is removed. The edges of the incision are pulled together and sutured, creating a tighter, higher breast. The areola and nipple are recentered. If the areola is quite large and greatly distorted by the procedure, it too, can be reduced.

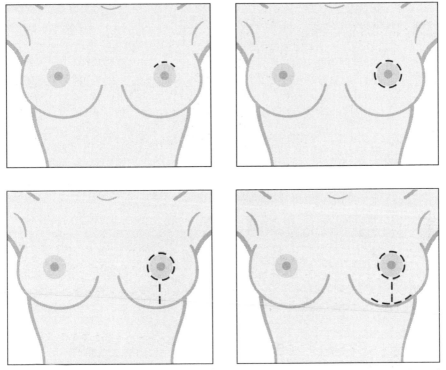

Depending on the amound of skin to be removed and the surgeon's preferred technique, a breast lift can be accomplished with a crescent incision (top left), a periareolar incision (top right), a lollipop incision (bottom left), or an anchor incision (bottom right).

Recovery. Your breast will be bruised for a few days and the swelling may last up to six weeks or more. You'll progress to a soft support bra within seven to 10 days; you musn't lift anything over five pounds during this time, or until your surgeon says it's okay to do so. For the next two or three weeks, you'll need to wear a sports bra around the clock. Most women can return to work within two weeks and resume full activities in three weeks.

Potential complications. Your nipple and breast may be numb for six weeks or more or until the swelling goes down. Some women experience this numbness for up to a year, and in rare cases, permanently.

As your breast settles, your nipples may be off-center or positioned unevenly and may require minor surgery to improve symmetry. This procedure shouldn't affect your ability to breastfeed, because the milk ducts generally aren't disturbed.

Breast lifts aren't permanent. Eventually, gravity, age, or other factors will cause them to sag again.

Chapter 14

Final Touches: Creating the Nipple and Areola

Years may wrinkle the skin,
but to give up enthusiasm wrinkles the soul.
– Samuel Ullman

When your breast mound has healed and dropped into its final position, you're ready for the concluding reconstructive step: creating the nipple and areola. This does involve a bit more surgery, but it's minor compared to mastectomy and building the breast mound. A small flap of skin—a mini tissue flap—is used to create the nipple. The surrounding skin is later tattooed a darker shade to create the areola. Your new nipple won't have any sensation, but it will look quite real.

Icing on the Cake

Recreating the nipple is a physical and psychological milestone. It completes the restoration of your missing breast, and for many women, signals an end to the breast cancer experience.

Creating a nipple is the icing on the reconstruction cake, but not everyone likes icing. Emotionally, you might not want to face yet another procedure and may decide to skip nipple surgery altogether. Or perhaps you're concerned with the physical limitations of a reconstructed nipple: it's a permanent bump on the breast mound. Because it doesn't react to sensation, your new nipple won't change from flat to erect and back to flat again, as a natural nipple does.

If you have unilateral reconstruction, this means your new nipple will be standing at attention when your natural nipple isn't. With bilateral reconstruction, both nipples will always be raised. This is something to keep in mind when you're deciding how large you'd like your nipples to be. The "perfect" nipple is said to be three or four times wider than its projection from the breast.

Planning your procedure. The best time to discuss nipple reconstruction with your surgeon is during your initial consultation. Inquire about the technique he prefers. Ask him to describe the best and worst results you can expect and look at his before-and-after photos. Be sure you are both clear about your desired size, shape, and projection.

Nipple reconstruction can be performed under local anesthesia in the surgeon's office. Your insurance company, however, may consider in-office procedures as cosmetic, rather than necessary, and cover related costs only if the nipple procedure is done in a hospital or surgical facility.

Building the Nipple

Traditionally, surgeons used skin grafts from elsewhere on the body to reconstruct the nipple. Now most surgeons fashion a nodule from tissue on the breast mound. Another technique called nipple sharing uses part of a patient's opposite, healthy nipple. There's an obvious downside to this: the procedure may reduce or eliminate feeling, erogenous sensation, and the ability to breastfeed in the only fully-functional nipple a woman has left after mastectomy.

My surgeon tried to convince me to "finish the job," but nipples didn't seem important. That was four years ago, and I still don't regret my decision. If I change my mind, I can always have them added. – Carole

Wow! My new nipple is amazing! It matches my other nipple almost exactly. The only way it could be better is if it had feeling. – Karla

If you have unilateral reconstruction, your new nipple will be sized and positioned to closely match your natural nipple. Bilateral nipples are centered at the front of the breast mounds.

Skin grafts. Nipples can be rebuilt with grafts from the labia, inner thigh, or earlobe. The skin in these areas has more pigment than breast skin and produces a darker nipple. Unlike a flap, which has its own blood supply, a graft is dependent on reestablished blood flow on the breast. Excess skin from the end of the mastectomy scar or the reconstruction flap scar may also be used.

Skin that typically grows hair will do so when grafted to the breast. If the skin above your hip is used, for example, your new nipple will sprout hair. Although it's possible to remove hair follicles from the skin graft before forming the nipple, this can be difficult. One solution is to have electrolysis on the new nipple or pluck the hairs yourself. It's worth discussing with your surgeon before the procedure.

Flaps. Nipples created with flaps from the reconstructed breast mound are more reliable. They are less likely to flatten or lose their shape because some of the underlying fat is used with the island of skin. There are many ways to do this. The most common is the skate flap. Other techniques include the star flap, bell flap, fishtail flap, and omega flap; all named for the shape of the incision made.

The flap pattern is first marked on the breast. The surgeon makes the incisions, freeing a small portion of skin from the breast. He pulls and twists the ends of skin to form a nipple-shaped nodule, and then stitches it closed. Nipples are made up to 40 percent larger than the desired final size to compensate for shrinkage during the first year.

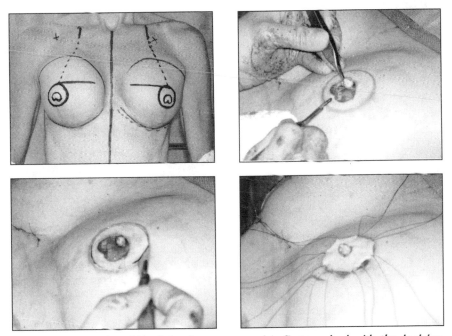

The skate flap: The skin of the breast mound is first marked with the incision lines (top left). The skin is excised along the markings, lifted, and formed into a nipple (top right). The areolar outline is excised (bottom left), and filled in with a circle of skin from somewhere else on the body (bottom right).

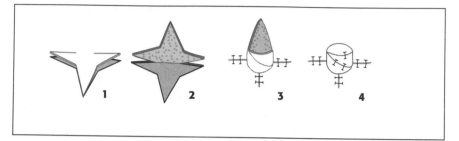

Nipple flaps are made with tissue from the breast mound. When a star flap is created, for example, the skin is excised along three sides (1) and lifted (2). The two lateral points are wrapped around the top (3), then tucked down and sutured in place (4).

Recovery. Antibiotic ointment is applied to protect the newly reconstructed nipple. For about two weeks, it will be covered with gauze or a small foam or plastic protective ring. The donor site will also have a light dressing.

Each nipple can be reconstructed in about an hour. No surgical drains are required after the operation. Any discomfort is usually mild (remember, there are no nerves in the new nipple) and can be managed with over-the-counter analgesics. If you have a skin graft, you may be sore for up to two weeks at the donor site.

You can wear a lightweight bra while the nipple is healing, but nothing that applies too much pressure. You should be able to return to your normal activities, including work, within three or four days. No matter which technique is used to create your nipple, it will need a healthy blood supply to survive. Don't smoke or use aspirin or other blood-thinning medications for a few weeks before and after your nipple procedure. Avoid caffeine products and keep the nipple dry during that period.

Adding the Areola

Once the nipple is formed, the surrounding areola is created with a skin graft or a tattoo. When a graft is used, a circular patch of skin is excised from the inside thigh or below the hip. If the skin graft is too light, it can be tattooed to add more color.

Tattooing the skin around the nipple is a less invasive way to simulate an areola. Although tattooing the skin only adds color—it doesn't create texture or projection—it can create a very realistic result. One advantage of tattooing is that it provides control over the amount of pigment. If you don't like what you see, you can change it. It's easy work to enlarge or recolor a tattoo, but you can't easily make it smaller or lighter. Tattoing the areola also camouflages the tiny incisions from the skin graft.

Who does the tattoo? Tattooing is an in-office procedure. Some surgeons do it themselves. Others refer patients to a different surgeon or a local tattoo artist. Always get approval from your insurance company if someone other than your reconstructive surgeon will tattoo your new breast. No matter who adds the pigment, ask about their specific experience with reconstructive breast tattoos. Review before-and-after photos of their work and speak with their previous patients.

In my surgeon's office, my tattoo color seemed much too brown. But after it faded in a couple of weeks, it was very nice. – Zoe

I was disappointed when my surgeon referred me to a local tattoo artist. I certainly wasn't comfortable baring my breast to yet another stranger! But the artist was very kind and specialized in reconstruction tattoos. He put me at ease and did a lovely job. – Lynne

Choosing your colors. Before your tattoo, you'll select the shade you want. Your doctor will give you a color chart with many different hues of beige, brown, tan, pink, rose, and other colors. After unilateral mastectomy, you can match the color swatch to your natural nipple. If you have bilateral reconstruction, some surgeons recommend matching the color to your lips. If you'd like your reconstructed areolas to be the same shade as your pre-mastectomy breasts, select your tattoo color *before* your mastectomy. Alternatively, ask your surgeon for a copy of your pre-op photos; you can use them as a reference.

Blending two or more shades sometimes produces the most natural result. You might need to combine a bit of rose with brown, or mix beige and pink, to get the shade you want. Choose a shade somewhat darker than your final color—tattooed areolae often fade as much as 40 to 50 percent. Pigment applied in layers over two or three sessions creates a more even coloration with less fading.

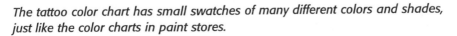

The tattoo color chart has small swatches of many different colors and shades, just like the color charts in paint stores.

How it's done. Whoever does your tattoo will first swab your breast with alcohol and mark the outline of the areola. Be sure to look at the markings in a mirror before tattooing begins. If you're trying to match your other breast, the outlined area should be same size and shape as your natural areola. If both breasts are to be colored, be sure the markings are centered on your new breast mounds and that you're happy with the placement before the tint is applied.

A thick layer of the pigment is spread inside the marked area. Don't be shocked when you first see the color. It's shiny and looks like thick frosting. Once under the skin, it fades to a more subtle shade.

The color is applied by a fine needle powered by an electric pump. As the needle moves over the marked area, it punches color under the skin. You'll feel more pressure or tingling than pain, because of the lost sensation in your breast. Some women report pain or discomfort elsewhere in the chest. Ask for a local anesthetic if you've regained some feeling in the front of your breast or just want to be on the safe side.

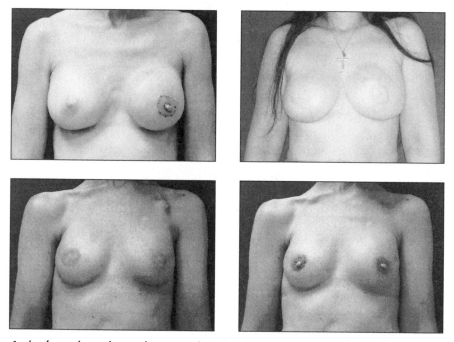

A nipple and areola can be created to closely match the opposite breast (top left: left breast reconstruction). Some areolar skin grafts must be tattooed to add color (top right: bilateral reconstruction). Others are darker (bottom left: bilateral reconstruction), but appear more natural after tattooing (bottom right: bilateral reconstruction).

In about half an hour, your tattooing is completed. Your new nipple and areola will be covered with antibiotic ointment and gauze. There's usually no down time from tattooing. You should be fine and can return to work the same day. You may need to go back for another tattooing to darken the area, create the desired shade, or fill in any uneven spots.

Your doctor will want you to keep the tattooed area dry for a few days. Temporarily, it's back to sponge baths or sitting in the tub. In four or five days, a scab will form over the tattooed area. Take care not to rub, scrub, or pick at it. That may create a splotchy, uneven color. Chlorine can prematurely fade your tattooed color; avoid swimming pools and hot tubs for about six weeks until your nipples are fully healed.

Questions for Your Plastic Surgeon

- How will you create my nipple and areola?
- How many of these procedures have you done?
- Where will the procedure be performed, and how long will it take?
- Will I have an anesthetic?
- Will I have any down time from the procedure?
- How closely will my new nipple and areola match my opposite breast?
- Where will I have scars, and how conspicuous will they be?
- Will I need a tattoo? Who will do it?
- What if I'm not satisfied?

Problems and Solutions

Serious problems rarely occur with new nipples. Most complications involve cosmetic flaws, which may require additional minor procedures to correct.

Nipple collapse. A reconstructed nipple may lose projection and collapse within a few weeks or few years of surgery. This happens more frequently when a skin graft is used or when the skin at the donor site is thin. Radiation, scar tissue, and trauma can also cause a nipple to flatten. The solution is to repeat the procedure using a flap technique, or insert additional tissue or cartilage under the graft. Sometimes synthetic skin is inserted in the nipple to keep it from collapsing.

Poor position. The best way to avoid off-center nipples and areolae is to wait until your reconstructed breast is fully healed before having nipple surgery. If you're going to be tattooed, be sure you're satisfied with the pre-tattoo markings before the color is applied.

Non-Surgical Alternatives

If you decide not to have your nipples reconstructed, tattooing a smaller dark circle in the areola creates the illusion of a nipple. It's not as realistic as a three-dimensional nipple, but it's an acceptable option for many women.

You can also use lifelike artificial semi-erect nipple prostheses that stick onto your reconstructed breast. If you have one healthy breast and one reconstructed breast, this will give you an even appearance. Check the suppliers mentioned in Chapter 2.

From Prep to Post-Op

Chapter 15

Preparing for Your Surgery

A woman is like a tea bag.
You never know how strong she is
until she gets into hot water.

– Eleanor Roosevelt

By now, you've done all your research and seen all the photos. You've talked to your surgeon about your reconstruction; how it will be done and what to expect. Your surgery date is circled in red on the kitchen calendar. There's a lot to be done before then, and now's the time to start.

Countdown: Four Weeks to Surgery

Here's a list of the activities you can expect within a month of your operation.

Finalize payment arrangement. You should have written confirmation of your health insurer's payment authorization or have a payment plan in place.

Take good care of yourself. Surgery is an assault on the body and its defenses, and fatigue is one of the most common side effects of general anesthesia. As a cancer patient, you've dealt with many stressful decisions and issues. All this takes a toll on your physical strength. If you've also undergone chemo or radiation, your resiliency has been further weakened.

Now, more than ever, your body needs special care to prepare for surgery and improve your ability to recover. This is no time to try that new diet. Eat a balanced diet with plenty of lean protein—meats, poultry, fish, and low-fat or non-fat dairy products are good sources— fiber, fruits, and vegetables. Drink plenty of fluids; avoid alcohol. Take a multivitamin with minerals.

If you'll be giving blood for your operation, it's important to increase your iron intake before and after surgery. Iron-rich foods including liver, tofu, beans, eggs, and lean poultry and meats are better sources than supplements, which can cause constipation. Vitamin C boosts iron absorption. Drink eight ounces of orange juice or other fortified juice with your meals. Avoid coffee, tea, sodas, or other products with caffeine, which can block iron absorption.

Exercise moderately for at least 30 minutes a day. Enjoy a walk with the dog or try a new exercise video. Get eight hours of sleep each night.

Prepare emotionally. Many well-documented studies show people who are emotionally prepared for surgery have less pain and heal sooner. Deal with stress and anxiety proactively. Try deep breathing exercises, yoga, or a walk around the block. Relaxation tapes and positive visualization are also helpful. *Prepare for Surgery, Heal Faster,* by Peggy Huddleston, is an excellent resource.

Stop smoking. You must stop smoking three to four weeks before and after your surgery. If you continue to smoke, your surgery will be delayed. This could be the push you need to quit for good.

Stop taking certain medications or supplements. Your surgeon will tell you which, if any, medications, vitamins, herbs, or supplements you should avoid. Products containing aspirin or ibuprophen can thin the blood and inhibit clotting—something you definitely don't want when you are going to have an operation. Taking any or all of these products is a no-no at least two weeks before and after surgery. You might be surprised to know how many over-the-counter products this includes:

Aspirin	Advil	Alka-Seltzer	Anacin	Aspergum
Bufferin	Coricidin	Darvon	Dristan	Ecotrin
Emprin	Excedrin	Fiorinal	Midol	Motrin
Naprosyn	Nuprin	Percodan	Sine-Aid	Sine-Off

When in doubt, read the label. Use Tylenol for relief from a headache, sore muscles, or other minor conditions. If you're taking Coumadin or other blood thinners, your doctor may request a blood test just prior to your surgery to make sure your blood clots sufficiently.

Your hormone replacement therapy may be a culprit too, potentially promoting bleeding and swelling. Consult with your gynecologist if your surgeon recommends you temporarily stop taking hormones until you've recovered from reconstruction.

Two Weeks before Surgery

Pre-op testing. About two weeks before your operation, your surgeon will explain the pre-op procedures and instructions. He'll also prescribe post-surgical pain medication and antibiotics, and give you the warranty information for your implants. He'll order routine preliminary tests, including:

- A Complete Blood Count (CBC) test to check your red and white blood cell counts.
- A chest X-ray.
- An electrocardiogram (EKG) to check your heart rhythm.

These are standard, precautionary tests to make sure you're healthy enough for surgery. Your surgeon may order additional tests, depending on your overall health and reconstructive procedure.

Understand the process and your instructions. Your surgeon will probably discuss the following issues with you before your operation. Be sure to ask him if he doesn't.

Questions for Your Surgeon before Your Operation

- How long will my surgery last?
- How long will I stay in the hospital?
- Do I need to buy a special post-operative bra or camisole?
- What medications will I need at home, and how long will I take them?
- How long until I may shower or bathe?
- When will I be able to drive?
- When will my stitches be removed?
- When is my next office appointment after I'm discharged from the hospital?

Donate blood. The surgeon will explain your option to provide blood, in case you need a transfusion during surgery. This is very unlikely with mastectomy and implant surgeries, but you may be asked to donate one or two units as a precaution if you're scheduled for an abdominal flap.

Shop for post-op garments. Your surgeon will tell you if you should bring a special sports bra or compression garment to the hospital, or what you should wear over your breasts in the weeks following your surgery. Buy something with a front closure. Bring this up if he doesn't mention it—you won't feel like wandering through the mall after your surgery. This is also a good time to shop for comfy camisoles, loose clothing or pretty new pajamas (with zippers or buttons in the front). Underwear a size or two larger than you normally wear is a good idea if you're having an abdominal flap.

Fill prescriptions. Your surgeon will prescribe pain medication and antibiotics for you to take once you return home. If you think you'll have trouble getting to sleep the night before your surgery, request a mild sleeping medication. This is also a good time to refill any other medications you routinely take, so you'll have an ample supply during your recovery. You may not be able to press down enough to open childproof lids after surgery; consider asking the pharmacist for a different type lid.

One Week to Go

Pre-admitting information. Many hospitals like to take care of the admitting information before the patient arrives. Someone from the staff may call you a few days before your surgery to obtain the necessary data.

Pamper yourself. Now is a great time to get your hair cut and colored, have a manicure (no polish or artificial nails), or engage in your favorite self-indulgent behavior. Have lunch with friends. Finish that big project at home or work. Go shopping. Take your kids on a trip. Have fun. Consider having your underarms and legs waxed—you won't be able to shave for two or three weeks after surgery.

Notify your surgeon of any health problems. Between now and your surgery date, notify your surgeon's office if you get a cold, fever, infection, allergy, cold sores, or other health problem, no matter how minor it may seem. Your surgery may have to be rescheduled if there is risk of infection, but it's always better to be safe than sorry.

Catch up, stock up. A little preparation now will make things easier on you and your family when you come home from the hospital.

- Shop for groceries and stock up on fresh fruits and vegetables, juices, and items that are easy for someone else to prepare. Or cook up a batch of reheatable meals and stock the freezer. This is especially important if you don't have someone who can shop and cook for you during your recovery. Have small bags of ice or frozen food on hand to wrap in a towel and apply to discourage swelling. Don't forget supplies for your pets.

- Buy a thermometer, if you don't already have one. It will come in handy if you think you might have a fever.

- Stock up on film and check your camera batteries if you'd like to keep a photo journal of your recovery, as many women do.

- Clean your house or have it cleaned before you go into the hospital. You won't be able to sweep, dust, or push a vacuum for a while.

- Catch up on the laundry.

Prepare for recovery. Do as much as possible now to get ready for your recovery.

- List errands other family members will need to take care of, such as paying bills, going to the dry cleaners, picking up the kids, and changing the litter box.

- Make a contact list of telephone numbers or e-mail addresses of friends and family who should be notified after surgery and kept posted on your recovery.

- Let others help. Line up volunteers to take care of the kids (for at least 48 hours after your surgery), the pets, and do errands for you. It's also wonderful when friends coordinate the delivery of meals for you and your family while you're recovering and unable to cook.

- Arrange for someone to drive you to the hospital and take you home. You'll also need someone to stay with you for at least the first 48 hours.

- Arrange your nightstand with all the things you'll need, including pain medication, TV/video/DVD remote, books and magazines, tissues, lotion, telephone (if you want it). Baby wipes are handy for the times when you just don't feel like getting up—although getting up and to the bathroom is good for you. You'll also want to have water and saltines or graham crackers handy for taking pain medication in the middle of the night. Keep a journal and pen or a small tape recorder handy if you're inclined to document your thoughts while you're recovering.

- Reposition bathroom and kitchen items on counters where you can get to them easily without reaching. If you are having an abdominal flap, do the same with items positioned under cabinets and on low shelves so you won't need to bend down to get them.

- Ask friends not to call for a few days after you come home from the hospital. Having the phone ring just when you drop off to sleep can be very disrupting. If you feel like talking, you can always call them. You can also turn down the ringer or unplug the phone so you won't be disturbed.

The Day Before Surgery

Remove all nail polish and artificial nails. The nails of your fingers and toes should be au naturel when you go into surgery. Your anesthesiologist will monitor them to determine if you're getting enough oxygen during surgery.

Get some extra pillows. Unless you've had a gluteal flap, you'll be sleeping on your back with your upper body elevated, so you'll need lots of pillows on the bed. (Chapter 17 provides tips for sleeping comfortably.)

Relax in your favorite way. See a movie with friends, have dinner with your family or favorite person, or put on some music and stretch out in a warm bath.

Wash with antibacterial soap. Twice daily for two days before your operation, wash your entire chest, sides, and underarms with Dial, Hibiclens, or other over-the-counter antibacterial soap. This helps eliminate bacteria on the skin and reduces the possibility of infection. If you're having flap reconstruction, thoroughly wash the donor site and surrounding area as well.

Decide what you'll wear to and from the hospital. Loose-fitting shirts or tops that button in the front are best—you won't be able to pull anything over your head. Wear sweatpants, pajama bottoms, or other loose, comfy pants. If you're having abdominal surgery, baggy pants or something that won't rest directly on your incision is helpful. Wear slippers or flat-heeled shoes.

Pack a small overnight bag. Take moisturizer, lip gloss, toothbrush and toothpaste, floss, hair brush or comb, eyeglasses (you can't wear contact lenses during your operation) and any other essentials. Don't take a nightgown. The hospital will want you to wear the one they provide for easier access to your tubes and drains. The hospital will also provide slippers and a robe, but you can bring your own if you wish.

It's also nice to pack a battery-operated portable CD player and your favorite music or books-on-tape, particularly if you'll be in the hospital for several days. Don't forget a sports bra if your surgeon recommended one, your insurance card, and any paperwork the surgeon asked you to bring to the hospital. If you'd like to have a record of your hospital experience, bring a small tape recorder or journal. Many women, particularly those who are used to journaling, find it gratifying to record their thoughts.

Pack a special bag for your husband or whoever will accompany you to the hospital. They'll be spending long hours in the waiting room. Include water, a snack, something to read, and a list of family and friends to notify after your surgery. Be sure to charge the cell phone or pack plenty of change for the pay phone.

Leave all valuables at home. Don't take anything you don't need. Leave cash, credit cards, your purse, wallet, and all jewelry, including wedding rings, earrings, and watches, at home.

Leave all medications at home. There's no need to bring prescribed medications to the hospital. Your surgeon will order all the medicine you'll need during your hospital stay, including any prescribed by other doctors.

Talk to your anesthesiologist. If he hasn't already done so, your anesthesiologist will call to ask questions about your general health, allergies, and any past reactions you may have had to anesthesia. If you were nauseous after a prior general anesthetic, for example, he may include an anti-nausea medication with your anesthesia.

Eat a light dinner. Don't eat or drink anything, including water, after midnight or the cutoff time advised by your anesthesiologist. Surgery is performed on an empty stomach to avoid the possibility of vomiting. If your surgery is scheduled for the afternoon, your anesthesiologist may approve Gatorade, water, cranberry or apple juice, or other clear beverage. Always inform your doctor or anesthesiologist if you eat or drink anything after the advised cutoff period.

Make love, if you feel like it. Many women question whether this is okay the night before surgery, but there's no medical reason to avoid sex, if you're so inclined. It's going to be several weeks before you'll be doing this again. It may even help calm your nerves.

It's Reconstruction Day

Shower and wash your hair. Wash all surgical areas again with antibacterial soap. This will be the last chance to wash your hair for several days after your operation. Don't shave your armpits or legs; any nick or cut may invite infection, and your surgery may be rescheduled.

Don't wear makeup. Your natural skin tone is an indication of adequate circulation.

Talk to someone. Chat with your kids, your spouse, your significant other, or best friend. It will help to quiet any concerns they're having. It will help you too.

Leave little notes. Tuck loving encouraging notes under your kids' pillows so they'll have a message from you even when you're not there.

Try to relax. It's natural to be nervous before surgery. But you can take steps to calm your thoughts and fears. Enjoy your morning shower or bath. Lie flat on the floor, close your eyes, breathe deeply, and focus on the most positive, beautiful thoughts you can—a gloriously happy time, a romantic vacation, or giggling with your children. Visualize a peaceful, happy post-operative you.

Chapter 16

In the Hospital

*One doesn't discover new lands without consenting
to lose sight of the shore for a very long time.*

– André Gide

Who doesn't get the jitters just walking into a hospital? It's a place we associate with the sick and ailing. Knowing what to expect once you're within those sanitized walls can help calm your fear of the unknown.

Admitting and Pre-Op

The hospital will want you to arrive two to three hours before your surgery. Once there, you'll be asked to review and sign a mountain of paperwork, including:

- A general information form listing your name, address, health insurance information, surgeon, primary care doctor, and next of kin.

- A questionnaire about your medical history. You'll be asked about your allergies, previous surgeries, whether you smoke or not, and other similar information. By this time, you will have gone over this information several times for various doctors, but this is an important precaution. The hospital doesn't want to give you Demerol for your pain if it makes you sick, or serve you strawberries if they give you hives.

- Notification you've received a copy of the Patient's Bill of Rights (provided when you are admitted), a document that outlines the hospital's responsibilities and your rights.

- A surgical consent form identifying the procedure to be performed and the name of your surgeon. Be sure you read this and verify the information. Signing the form also means you understand the potential risks of the operation.

- A power of attorney form, giving a person you designate authority to make financial and other decisions on your behalf, if necessary. This can unnerve the calmest of women, but don't fear. It's a formality in the unlikely event something untoward happens to you during surgery.

- A release of negligence, meaning you won't hold the hospital responsible if something goes wrong. This doesn't mean you can't sue if something does go amiss.

- Authorization for the hospital to provide you with blood from its supply, if necessary, unless you're donating your own blood before surgery.

A nurse will show you to your room and ask you to change into a hospital gown. She will weigh you, take your blood pressure, and ask you to remove hearing aids, dentures, prosthetic limbs, contact lenses, or any other artificial apparatus before entering the operating room (OR).

While you are waiting. Your general surgeon (if you're having a mastectomy) and plastic surgeon will come by to chat with you before you enter the OR. If your plastic surgeon didn't mark the incision reference lines on your body the previous day, he'll draw them now.

> *I was so nervous the day of my surgery, I broke into a cold sweat. I remember wondering if I would be admitted for heart problems instead of reconstruction, because I could feel my heart hammering beneath my shirt.*
> *– Laney*

The anesthesiologist will stop by to introduce himself and review your medical history (again). He'll mix up a batch of custom anesthesia just for you, based on your weight, the length of your surgery, and any previous reactions you've had to anesthesia.

There's always a lot of waiting before surgery. Free to wander, your mind may go directly to uneasy. Breathe deeply. Concentrate on the positive aspects of your surgery. Mastectomy will remove your cancer, and reconstruction will restore your breast. Don't be a brave little soldier if it will make you feel better to discuss your fears with your doctors, your husband, family, or others who are in the hospital with you.

In the OR

It's showtime. When it's time for your surgery, you'll be taken to the OR on a gurney (a bed with wheels). In some private or small facilities you may simply walk in. Friends and family will be shown to the waiting room.

As soon as you enter the OR, you'll notice it's very bright and very cold. The temperature is deliberately kept low because lights in the room generate a lot of heat and the surgical staff wear several layers of clothing to protect from bacteria.

You'll be moved to the operating table, and the pre-surgery preparations begin. A nurse will cover you immediately with heated blankets. Small sensors will be stuck to your arms and legs to monitor your heartbeat, blood pressure, and the level of oxygen in your blood. You may be anxious, but not for long—you'll soon be fast asleep.

I began shivering as soon as I got into the operating room. I guess from nerves as much as the cold. A nurse immediately covered me with warm blankets. They felt wonderful and reassuring. – Sharon

You'll feel a small sting (similar to having your blood drawn) as the anesthesiologist inserts a thin needle into a vein inside your arm or on your hand. Through this intravenous (IV) tube, he'll administer a complex and precise anesthesia directly into your bloodstream. He may give you a sedative first. You'll be asleep before you can count to five.

After you're asleep. Once asleep, you'll receive pain medication, so you won't feel a thing during surgery. A surgical tube will be placed in your throat to help you breathe and a plastic tube called a *Foley catheter* will be inserted into your bladder to control your urine. A nurse will wash your chest and donor site with surgical disinfectant. If you're having a TRAM or DIEP flap, she will shave your pubic area. Then the rest of your body will be draped with sterile sheets, leaving only the surgical areas uncovered.

The technology of anesthesia has vastly improved in the past five to 10 years. It's an incredibly complex, yet precise practice. Yet when patients are asked what they fear most about surgery, most say it's the anesthesia. They're afraid they'll overdose or wake up during the operation in horrible pain. In fact, close monitoring by the anesthesiologist prevents either of these mishaps. He monitors your vital signs during the operation and carefully controls your level of consciousness, administering just enough sedative to keep you in a deep sleep. Not too much, not too little—just enough.

Many patients fear they'll talk in their sleep, divulging some deep, dark secret once they're under: announcing their crush on the gardener or confessing to the extra pint of chocolate Häagen-Dazs hidden behind the frozen peas. It's not likely. Others worry they'll embarrass themselves by urinating or defecating. Unless you're in the habit of doing that in your sleep at home, it's not likely to occur under anesthesia either.

The general surgeon begins your mastectomy as described in Chapter 4. The plastic surgeon then moves in to do the reconstruction.

A Peek into Post-Op

When your surgery is over, you'll be wheeled into the recovery room for about an hour. A nurse will carefully monitor your vital signs and make sure you're doing okay before taking you to your room. The recovery room is quite noisy. It can be disconcerting waking up to machines humming and beeping all around you. If you've had flap reconstruction, a surgical wire will be inserted into the new breast to monitor the blood flow. You'll be closely monitored in the intensive care unit overnight.

Your nurse will give you ice chips if your mouth feels dry, and warm blankets if you're chilled. You shouldn't be in pain, because you'll be given pain medication intravenously during your surgery. The nurse can give you additional pain medication if you need it and anti-nausea medicine if your stomach is upset. Visitors aren't allowed here, but your surgeon will go to the waiting room to let your loved ones know you're out of surgery.

In your room. Your head will feel very fuzzy for the next 24 to 48 hours, until the effects of the anesthesia wear off. Anesthesia suppresses the body's ability to function normally. The longer you're under its influence, the longer your body needs to recover.

You won't remember the operation. Your chest and donor site will be bandaged. You may be curious and perhaps anxious to see what's under there, but won't be able to until the dressing is removed in your doctor's office in a few days. Your bed will be angled to elevate your chest, so you'll be reclining in a semi-upright position. If you had abdominal surgery, the lower portion of the bed will be positioned to lessen tension on your incision.

The pain was hard to bear after my TRAM flap. My husband asked the hospital staff for permission to stay in my room beyond visiting hours. Having him there was a great comfort.
– Alice

Your room will have a call button or an intercom to summon your nurse whenever you need help. If you can't reach it easily, ask the nurse to bring it closer. An IV attached to your hand or arm will drip saline and antibiotics into your bloodstream. Your pain medication will also be administered through the IV, unless the hospital provides a self-medicating pain pump. The amount of medication is regulated, so you can't overdose.

The Foley catheter will still be in your bladder, so you won't have to get up or use a bedpan to urinate. Some women don't even feel the catheter. Others say it makes them feel they have to urinate when they don't. The catheter will be removed when you can walk to the bathroom on your own.

Typically, patients don't have bowel movements for three to five days following general anesthesia. Eating lightly will help to avoid a bloated feeling that can put pressure on an abdominal incision. Walking and drinking lots of fluid and fiber will help get you back on track. You can always ask the nurse for a laxative or stool softener, if needed. When you're able to eat and drink, the IV will be removed and you'll switch to oral medication.

Pressurized elastic stockings on your legs will help prevent blood clots until you're able to move around. You'll feel a gentle pressure as a pumping machine periodically compresses the stockings to mimic normal circulation. The machine is somewhat noisy, whooshing rather loudly with each pumping action.

You'll be very thirsty from the anesthesia and may have a sore throat from the breathing tube. Ask your nurse for water, juice, or throat lozenges. She will frequently check your temperature, blood pressure, pulse, and empty your surgical drains. She'll continue to administer pain medication (unless you have a pain pump) and antibiotics through your IV throughout the night.

The Day after Surgery

Anesthesia is hard on the lungs. A ventilating machine breathed for you while you were in surgery; now it is important to get your lungs back up to full capacity. This takes a bit of effort. At first, a small plastic tube inside your nose delivers oxygen. Your nurse will use a finger clamp called a *pulse oximeter* to periodically check the level of oxygen in your blood. When you're breathing well enough to inhale sufficient oxygen into your system, the tube will be removed.

A *triflow* unit will help strengthen your breathing. It's a plastic box divided into three separate chambers, each with a small ball. To use the triflow, you first exhale to expel the air in your lungs. As you inhale through the triflow mouthpiece, each ball rises independently and stays up as long as you hold your breath. Initially, it will be difficult to elevate even the first ball. Keep practicing two or three times each hour until you can keep all three balls at the top simultaneously. Don't skip this little exercise. Restoring lung strength is a very important part of your recovery.

Managing pain. To better understand the source of your pain, consider this: You know how annoying a paper cut can be—that affects only the top layer of skin. Your surgical incision is a paper cut magnified, slicing through skin, tissue, and muscle.

The trick to managing pain is keeping a constant, even flow of medication in your system. It typically takes 15 to 20 minutes for the medication to kick in, so ask for it before you're in excruciating pain. This is no time to be a tough guy—patients who control their pain heal faster than those who don't. Your nurse will administer pain medication every three or four hours, or as you need it.

Applying pressure to your incision, either internally or externally, will hurt. A sneeze or cough can feel like a grenade going off inside. Holding your hand or a pillow against your incision will help. Try to support your incisions in the same way when getting in or out of bed.

Circulation. Movement improves circulation, prevents fluid from settling in your lungs, and helps get your system back to normal. Carefully change position frequently while you're in bed. Flex your toes. Rotate your ankles and gently stretch your arms and legs. Move as many body parts as you can.

The sooner you're mobile, the sooner you'll be on the way to recovery. Getting out of bed for the first time will be an effort, particularly if you have an abdominal incision. But it is important to walk around and get your blood circulating, if just for a few moments. You'll be encouraged to get out of bed the day after your surgery. Start by sitting up carefully with the help of the nurse. Take a few steps around the room or walk to the bathroom. It will be exhausting, but the next day will be a little better. Get up every few hours and take a short stroll. Each time will be easier as you regain strength. It will easier to move around when you're not in pain; be sure you are amply medicated before you get out of bed. Once you're able to move around on your own, you'll be taken off the IV and switched to oral medication.

The Rest of Your Hospital Stay

Discharge. Although your health insurance may dictate the length of your stay, all bodily functions must be operating normally before you can leave the hospital. Contact your insurance company if you need to stay longer for any reason—if you don't feel well enough to go home or you develop an infection, for example.

Be sure you leave with the following:

- Instructions to care for your incisions.

- Directions for emptying and measuring the surgical drains.

- A list of warning signs for infection or other problems.

- Prescriptions for pain medication and antibiotics (if you didn't fill them before going into the hospital).

- Your surgeon's regular and out-of-hours contact information in case you need to reach him before your next appointment.

- A scheduled follow-up appointment with your surgeon.

When you're sure you've packed up everything you need and your surgeon has signed your discharge papers, a nurse will bring a wheelchair. For insurance reasons, patients aren't allowed to walk out of the hospital. She'll wheel you outside, and you're on your way home.

Recovery and
Beyond

Chapter 17

Back Home

*Today is the first day
of the rest of your life.*

– Abbie Hoffman

After surgery, your definition of a "good day" will change as you recover and regain strength. At first, a good day will involve simply finding a comfortable sleeping position. That will be redefined when you can stay awake, sit up, and have dinner with your family. Later, a good day will be one when you can lift your arms over your head or go the entire day without a nap. One day your cancer, treatment, reconstruction, and all the doctor appointments will be behind you. You'll go about your life and forget about your chest, just as you did before your surgery. And that will be a good day.

A Timetable for Healing

My doctor said she could tell I was a type A personality who would be impatient with recovery. She sternly cautioned me to get a stack of books and plan to do a lot of reading and relaxing and not much else. – Glory

Just three months after losing his legs in an accident on the track, world champion race car driver Alex Zanardi was up and walking on artificial limbs. Zanardi said of his recovery, "The good thing is that I've turned the first page of that book. Actually, I've finished the first chapter. All of the others are very, very short." Now that's a positive outlook on recovery. If you can view your own reconstruction with the same outlook—the worst is behind you—it will be easier to keep the end result in view.

Sleeping or resting will take up a large portion of your first few days at home. You'll be anxious to return to your normal routine, but don't rush your recovery. Give in to it and relax. Take advantage of the time to write in your journal, catch up on your reading, or watch favorite movies. As your body recuperates, so will your spirit. Don't be frustrated when you can't reach the top shelf or blow-dry your hair. Day by day, you will get better. Your functionality, strength, and range of motion will improve.

What You Will and Won't be Able to Do

10 THINGS YOU WON'T BE ABLE TO DO FOR A WHILE	10 THINGS YOU WILL BE ABLE TO DO
1. Shower	1. Chat with friends
2. Drive	2. Stroll in the yard
3. Laundry	3. Enjoy music
4. Vacuum	4. Watch TV or movies
5. Push-ups	5. Catch up on your photo albums
6. Lift your kids	6. Deliver kisses
7. Scratch your back	7. Read to your kids
8. Reach over your head	8. Plan your Christmas list
9. Slice a loaf of bread	9. Make a post-recovery to-do list
10. Open childproof bottle lids	10. Send e-mails or thank you cards to thoughtful family and friends

How long will it take to get back to normal? Recovery is such a personal matter, and it's different for everyone. A lot depends on your condition before surgery, the type of reconstruction you have, and how much you do to support rather than fight your body's recovery. Here's a general description of what you can expect. Your own recovery may move along faster or take a while longer.

Week 1. Whether you're home or still in the hospital, you'll feel very tired and perhaps lightheaded as your first post-operative week comes to a close. Pain medication throughout the day and night will help control your discomfort. Your chest will be bound tightly in a surgical bra or ACE bandage for several days. You may be more comfortable staying in your pajamas or nightgown, but walking for a few minutes every couple of hours is important. Begin the exercises your surgeon recommends or those listed in Chapter 18.

You may spend much of the time in bed, but you can dress (or not), take short walks down the hall or around the yard, work at the computer briefly, and take meals with the rest of the family. Your incisions should be kept dry, so you won't be able to shower for three to five days if you have implants, and five to 10 days after a flap reconstruction. In the meantime, you can take sponge baths or sit in a half-filled tub as long as you don't get your dressing or surgery area wet.

I always thought napping during the day was such a waste of time. After my surgery, I just gave into it. I kept a pile of books by bed. I would wake up, read a little, walk a little, then readjust my pillows and nod off again. How decadent! – Mona

Not showering doesn't mean you can't wash your hair. You probably won't really care for a few days, but if you can't wait to have clean hair—it's the most wonderful feeling—lean over the sink, cover your face with a towel, and have someone do the honors. Your clean hair may need to wait a while longer if you have an abdominal incision and can't manage this. To dry or style your hair, bend your head to the side to meet the dryer, brush, or comb, instead trying to raise your arm over your head.

You'll need to move slowly and carefully for a couple of weeks—no extensive reaching, stretching, pulling, or pressing movements—nothing that puts too much stress on your healing tissue. Avoid lifting anything over five pounds. It may hurt to lift your arms above chest level. Gentle walking and mild stretching are fine during this period. Arrange for someone else to do the cleaning, laundry, ironing, driving, or pick up the kids.

Your surgeon will see you in his office to check your incision and change your dressing. You'll need someone to drive you there and back home. He'll show you how to clean the incision to avoid infection. This is the first glimpse you'll have of your post-operative breast. That achievement is discussed later in this chapter. This is a good time to ask for a copy of your mastectomy pathology report and make sure a copy was sent to your oncologist.

If you have a lot of swelling, try icing your breast—15 minutes on, 15 minutes off—with ice cubes or a bag of frozen vegetables wrapped in a towel. Your breast must be supported until it heals, so you'll now begin to wear the sports bra or support garment your surgeon recommended.

Week 2. Most women find they can do more this week; it just takes longer and uses more energy. This is the time when many make the mistake of doing too much too soon. You won't feel like dancing yet, but you should feel better than the previous week. You're still recovering.

Never force yourself to do something before you're ready. Give yourself time to gradually get back into the swing of things. If you're ready to start weaning yourself from pain medication, lengthen the interval between doses.

Within a few days, you will reach two significant milestones in your recovery. Your drains will probably be removed (they'll remain if you have more than 30 cc of fluid in a 24-hour period) and—drum roll, please—you can finally take a nice, warm shower. You can't imagine how blissful this will feel. Be very careful, because you will still be weak. Remember your incision is still healing. Don't use harsh or scented soaps. If you have an adjustable spray, turn it to the gentlest setting and pat yourself dry. If you have an abdominal incision, it will be difficult to bend over. Once your doctor says it's okay to shower, a handheld showerhead or a child-size chair will make the task easier.

I was tired and fuzzy for a few days after my implant reconstruction, but I was okay as long as I took my pain pills. I was so much better by the second week, I decided to shop for groceries. What a mistake! I was utterly exhausted in 10 minutes. I couldn't push the cart one more step. I left it right in the middle of the cereal aisle, got back into my car, and had a good cry.
– Shelly

Add a minute or two more to your daily strolls, until you're walking for 20 to 30 minutes each time. Continue the recommended exercises, adding more as you heal. Move slowly and carefully. Allow yourself more time to do things you would otherwise rush through.

Week 3. By now you should be taking longer walks and staying up much, if not all, of the day. You may still need a nap or two, but you'll feel more alert and less fatigued.

Your surgeon will see you again to check your incision and make sure everything is healing properly. He'll probably also give you the okay to begin driving again. Do a test first: sit in a parked car and see how it feels to get in and out and turn the wheel. If it's too uncomfortable, wait another week. You can grocery shop, if you feel up to it, but ask someone to carry and unload your bags.

Until your chest heals, it will be difficult to execute pushing and pulling movements or any motion that puts pressure on your pectoral muscles or donor site incision. The surgeon will discuss any activities you should continue to avoid for awhile longer. You may return to sexual activity, as long as you and your partner are careful to be gentle and not put too much pressure on your incisions.

Cooking is my passion. During my recovery, I amassed a huge pile of new recipes from TV cooking shows I watched all day. I couldn't wait to try them. I didn't consider myself back to normal until the third week after my operation when I could get back into the kitchen. – Verna

Week 4. By now, you'll be back to most or all of your normal routine. If you've had a flap operation, it may take a week or two longer. If you smoke, you've been off cigarettes for six to eight weeks. What a great start to kick the habit! If you go back to smoking, don't resume until this week or when given permission by your doctor. If you had flap reconstruction and your new breast isn't sore, you can wear ordinary bras. Avoid underwire bras until your surgeon says it is okay (you don't want anything pushing into the tissue and restricting blood flow before the flap is adequately healed).

Phantom pains. As your nerves grow back, you may feel temporary shooting pains or a tickling, like when your foot goes to sleep. Some women also experience phantom pains: itching or tingling where the breast used to be. People who have lost an arm or a leg often report the same phenomenon. It's your brain continuing to send routine signals to the breast. In time, it will adjust to the fact that the breast and nerves are no longer there and the odd feelings will subside and disappear. In the meantime, if your reconstructed breast itches, scratching won't help, because you won't feel it. Try rubbing or scratching nearby, where you do have feeling.

My reconstructed breasts look fabulous, but I can't feel a thing. It's so weird! When I'm sitting down, I can lean forward and not even feel the edge of the table pressing into my new boobs. They could be on fire and I wouldn't know it! You get used to it after awhile. It doesn't mean you don't wish you had feeling, but you do get used to the numbness. – Angel

When to call your doctor. It's normal to have discomfort, soreness, and fatigue after surgery. Notify your doctor, however, if you experience any of the following symptoms of infection:

- Chills or a fever higher than 101 degrees.

- Persistent vomiting or nausea.

- Pale, blue, or cold fingers, toes, or nails.

- Pain that isn't controlled by your prescribed medication.

- Increased numbness, tingling, or swelling in your fingers.

- Redness, warmth, or excessive firmness around your incision.

- Excessive bleeding into your bandage or bleeding that doesn't stop when pressure is applied to the incision for 10 minutes. A cloudy discharge or foul odor may also indicate infection.

Managing Medication

Your doctor will prescribe pain medication and antibiotics after your surgery. Take the antibiotics on an empty stomach at regular intervals throughout the day until you've finished *all* of them. If they make you nauseous, don't take Maalox, Mylanta, Tums, or other antacids; they may negate the effectiveness of the antibiotics. Ask your surgeon for a different prescription instead.

Here are a few tips for managing your medications.

Take it if you need it. Studies show patients who manage their pain heal faster than those who don't. It's more effective to keep a level amount of pain medication in your system than wait until your pain becomes unmanageable.

Prevent nausea. Take pain pills with milk or food to prevent nausea. Antibiotics can be taken on an empty stomach or with food.

Be prepared during the night. In the first week or two after surgery, your pain will probably wake you up during the night. Time your pain pills so you have one just before you go to bed. Keep water or juice and a few saltine or graham crackers by your bed so you won't have to get up to take your medicine.

Combat constipation. Straining from constipation is often painful and puts added stress on abdominal incisions. Treating constipation pre-emptively will help. Increase your daily fiber intake with fruits, vegetables, whole grains, and legumes. Stay hydrated. Iron promotes constipation—if you take a multivitamin, use one without iron until your bowels are back to normal. Frequent walking will help restore your regularity. If your bowels refuse to cooperate, try an over-the-counter stool softener recommended by your doctor.

Don't drive while on pain medication. Pain medicines make you drowsy. Don't drive until you stop taking them.

Avoid alcohol. It exacerbates drowsiness from pain medication and can sometimes interfere with antibiotics.

Taper off. Take pain medication less frequently or take one pill instead of two when you begin to feel better. When you think you can tolerate something less, switch to extra-strength Tylenol.

Dealing with Drains

Many women consider surgical drains to be the most annoying aspect of their recovery. You'll be anxious to get rid of these pesky contraptions, but they promote healing by siphoning off fluids at the surgery sites. Just think what the post-surgical experience was before someone invented these drains: all that fluid you empty twice a day would otherwise be accumulating in your body, promoting swelling and delaying healing.

Until the early 1990s, patients stayed in the hospital until their drains were removed. Today, shorter hospital stays are emphasized, largely due to insurance pressures, but drains are easily managed at home.

Surgical drains are plastic bulbs with long tubing that is sutured under the skin at the incision sites. They're more irritating than painful, but they can be very sore where they enter the skin. Minimize soreness by immobilizing the drains as much as possible, so they don't pull on the small incision. Each drain has a plastic loop on top. Use it to pin the drain to the inside of your robe, shirt, belt loop, or waistband to hold it away from the incision and keep it from swinging or catching on furniture. Keep the point of entry clean by swabbing it every day with a Q-Tip dipped in a 50/50 solution of water and peroxide.

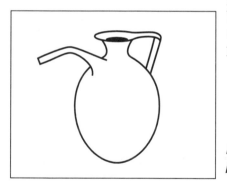

Fluids from the surgical site are collected in plastic surgical drains.

Drains are lumpy under clothing. Until they are removed, camouflage is your best fashion defense. Slip on an oversized shirt, vest, or sweater, and the drains will be hidden from view. You can stick them in your pants pocket for a short while if the tube isn't twisted or pinched and the bulb isn't flattened. Post-mastectomy garments like the Softee camisole have built-in pockets for surgical drains. When your drains come out, you can remove the pockets and have a soft everyday camisole. Find these special garments at your local mastectomy shop. Another clever garment, designed by a woman who has been through mastectomy, is the Marsupial Pouch (800-825-4325 or www.dermasciences.com). It's a terrycloth belt with an attachable pouch to hold surgical drains at the chest or abdomen.

Emptying the drains. You should empty the drains and measure the contents twice a day, 12 hours apart, at the same time each day. You may need to empty them more frequently if they fill up. Before you leave the hospital, a nurse will show you how to do this and provide a measuring cup and a log to record the amount of fluid collected each day. Here's what you'll do:

1. Wash your hands thoroughly with soap and water before and after handling drains.

2. Unpin the drain from your clothing.

3. Open the top of the drain bulb and empty the contents into the measuring container provided by the hospital. Be sure to squeeze the bulb to empty it completely. Note the color and characteristics of the fluid. Initially it will be bloody, then yellow, and finally clear. Notify your doctor if the fluid is cloudy, milky, or foul-smelling; any of these conditions may indicate infection.

4. Squeeze the empty bulb again to expel the air, and close the plug. This creates the suction necessary to remove fluids from the incision. Repin the drain to your clothing.

5. Record the amount of fluid on the log provided by the hospital. Once the level of fluid drops below 30 ccs (about two tablespoons) in a 24-hour period, your surgeon will remove the drains.

Those drains were the worst part of my reconstruction. One drain wouldn't be so bad, but I had four: one at each breast and two in my abdomen. One day the tubing caught on a doorknob as I walked by. It yanked sharply against the incision. Ouch!
– Michele

Sample Drain Log				
DATE	DRAIN 1	DRAIN 2	DRAIN 3	TOTAL
June 10/6am	5	30	30	65
June 10/6 pm	10	20	20	50
June 11/6 am	15	35	30	80
June 11/6 pm	10	35	30	75
June 12/6 am	0	50	20	70
June 12/6 pm	5	25	18	48
June 13/6 am	5	28	10	43
June 13/6 pm	3	15	14	32
June 14/6 am	1	10	9	20

6. Flush the fluids down the toilet.

7. Repeat the process with each of the other drains. Wash your hands again.

If a bloodclot clogs up the tube, try clearing it: with one hand, hold the tube where it enters your skin. Pinch the tube with your other hand to break up the clot. If that doesn't work, slide your fingers down the tubing away from your body to dislodge the blockage. You may have to repeat this a few times before it works. Notify your doctor if you can't dislodge the clot.

Removing the drains. When it's time to remove the drains, your surgeon will first snip the suture, then quickly yank the tubing out of the skin. You won't feel any discomfort if you take a big breath and forcibly exhale as he pulls the tube out.

Tips for an Easier Recovery

Much of your recovery depends on your own actions. First and foremost, be relentless in taking care of yourself. Your priority has to be you—not the job, the kids, or anyone else. You can't expect to come home from the hospital and immediately get back up to normal speed. Napping or just resting during the day when you feel tired is important. You needn't treat yourself like an invalid. Just don't overdo. The more things you do within your range of motion, the better.

The art of sleeping comfortably. Rest and sleep give your body time to direct its resources to healing. Finding a comfortable sleeping position once you get home can be a challenge. You need to sleep in a semi-upright position, as you were in the hospital. This keeps fluids from accumulating in your chest and makes getting out of bed easier. Sleeping in this position may be a bit strange at first, particularly if you're used to sleeping on your stomach or side. Many women find it more comfortable to sleep in a recliner during recovery. The chair is easily repositioned and it's easier to get in and out of than a bed.

One way to sleep comfortably in bed is to make a nest of pillows. First position a firm pillow against the headboard or wall—a body pillow with arm extensions or a sofa cushion works well—then arrange several pillows at an angle in front to serve as a backrest. Reposition the pillows until you get a comfortable arrangement. Place a pillow under your knees. Or lean your upper torso against several pillows behind you, and settle your lower torso and legs on another pillow perpendicular to the others. Elevate your surgery-side arm on a pillow or rolled-up towel to take pressure off your chest.

If you have a back or gluteal incision, sleep with your weight more to the unoperated side. Try elevating your buttock with a soft buckwheat pillow that conforms to your shape.

Getting into bed. Be very careful getting in and out of bed. Those simple movements we take for granted each morning and night will now be difficult. Think about how you're going to move before you actually do. First sit on the edge of the bed, and then swing your legs up. Cover the reconstructed breast with one arm and leverage your position with the other. Move up the bed by scooting your behind from side to side until you're reclining against the pillows. This is also the perfect reading posture.

My husband slept in our guest room for six weeks after my reconstruction. It was the only time in our marriage we've slept apart, but it helped. He wasn't afraid of rolling into me, yet he was close enough to hear me if I needed something during the night.
– Sylvia

Getting out of bed. After unilateral reconstruction, carefully roll out of bed on the healthy side and use your unaffected arm to leverage yourself into a sitting position. If you've had bilateral reconstruction, use your legs and abdominal muscles to first bring yourself into a sitting position at the edge of the bed. Swing your legs over the side. Plant your feet on the floor and slowly straighten your knees until you're standing.

Using an aromatherapy eye pillow and having white noise in the background helped me sleep on my back. My surgeon also prescribed a mild sleeping pill. – Sue

Entry and exit get trickier if you have an abdominal incision. You'll need someone to help you. Hold one arm over your chest and the other over your abdomen. If your bedroom is upstairs, consider sleeping on the main floor until you can navigate the stairs.

Oh, your aching back. Sleeping exclusively on your back and spending so much time in bed can give you a backache. Carefully and gently stretch your back to keep it limber and ward off discomfort. Do isometric exercises in bed, first contracting the muscles along the spine, then releasing them in very small, concentrated movements. Shrug your shoulders and roll your neck gently from side to side. When you're out of bed, stand straight while you flex your spine, as if you're pushing it against a wall, and then pull it back towards you. Do this several times a day.

Diet and nutrition. It's not unusual to gain weight during recovery. You'll be exercising less and may be eating more treats than you normally do, but now is not the time to diet. Your body will heal faster if you give it the balanced nutrition it needs. Indulge in moderation. Ask friends who provide meals to bring salads or nutritious entrées instead of cakes, cookies, or other high-fat foods. Eat sensibly and drink plenty of non-alcoholic fluids.

Recovery fashion. When your hospital dressings are removed, you'll need to wear something with adequate support and compression around the clock for a few weeks. If your surgeon doesn't recommend a particular garment, wear snug sports bras or specially designed surgical tops, like the Surgi-Bra (800-927-5568 or www.goldainc.com). Once your drains come out and you no longer need quite as much support, nylon or tricot camisoles with bra linings are very nice.

Seeing Your New Breasts for the First Time

It's not unusual to have conflicting feelings about seeing your new breast. On one hand, you'll be expectant and hopeful, waiting to see the outcome of several months of surgery, recovery, and waiting. You may feel anxious, fearing what you'll see as you look down at your chest. The reconstruction photos you have seen up to this point mean nothing. This is personal. This is your breast, not someone else's.

When I first saw my reconstructed breasts, I burst into tears. They were horrible! My doctor smiled and said my two little ugly ducklings would grow up to be beautiful swans. He was right. Nine months later, when I look at my breasts now it is hard to imagine they had such an ugly beginning.
– Holly

While most women react positively to reconstruction, some find themselves a bit at odds with their new breast. It won't feel or look like your natural breast. A breast created with flap reconstruction will be bruised and swollen. It may look pretty awful. If you've had a delayed reconstruction, your mastectomy incision will be a line of angry red stitches. If you have expanders, you'll see a baby breast mound with its first fill of saline.

Don't be surprised if your surgeon proclaims your breasts to be beautiful. Being far more used to this than you, he's able to see beyond the swelling and redness to see how your breast will ultimately look.

Remember you're a work in progress. This isn't what you'll look like several months or a year from now when you're fully healed and your scars have faded. You've suffered a very personal loss. Give yourself time to come to grips with it, maybe even grieve for it, if that feels right. Recovery is temporary. Hang in there, and know the worst is behind you.

Chapter 18

Building Strength and Flexibility with Exercise

If we could give every individual the right amount of nourishment and exercise, not too little and not too much, we would have found the safest way to health.

– Hippocrates

Exercising moderately for just 30 minutes a day enhances physical and mental well-being. It clears the mind, increases energy, controls weight, and improves overall health. Exercising before your reconstruction can help your body weather the stress of surgery. When pain and contracting scar tissue impair range of motion during recovery, restorative movements stimulate circulation and restore flexibility.

This chapter introduces exercises you can do before and after your operation. Your surgeon may recommend other movements. Always obtain his permission before beginning any exercise after reconstruction. Perform all movements gently and never to the point of pain. Move smoothly and with awareness.

Before Your Surgery

Four weeks or more before your surgery, begin strengthening your shoulders, arms, and chest. If you're going have TRAM or DIEP reconstruction, add sit-ups, stomach crunches, and other exercises to strengthen your abdominal muscles.

Aerobic exercise. Walking, swimming, dancing, and other aerobic exercises strengthen your lungs and heart, and boost your immune system.

Strength training. Lifting mild weights builds and tones muscle. You can also do push-ups, sit-ups, or other similar exercises, using your own body weight as resistance.

Stretching. Any good stretching program is beneficial after surgery. Regularly stretching the muscles increases flexibility, resilience, and range of motion. Yoga is particularly restorative, because it does all this and increases blood flow as well. Done daily, yoga poses can also relieve post-operative pain and discomfort. Always start slowly and learn from a qualified instructor. Check with yoga studios, your local gym, or the YWCA for nearby classes. Breast cancer survivor and yogi Susan Rosen has an easy-to-follow regimen on her video designed especially for breast surgery patients: "Yoga and the Gentle Art of Healing, A Journey of Recovery after Breast Cancer" (858-481-3912 or www.yogajoyofdelmar.com).

Deep breathing. Our bodies breathe reflexively. We don't have to think about breathing for it to occur. Consciously inhaling and exhaling, however, expands the lungs, bringing more oxygen into the body. When done correctly, deep breathing clears the mind and offers new perspective. It's a wonderfully effective way to restore calm after a stressful day or counter pre-surgery jitters.

Make a point of breathing deeply several times each day. You don't need any special equipment. Do it while watching TV or when you're stopped at a traffic light. Or lie on your back with one hand on your abdomen and the other on your chest. Slowly breathe in as much air as you can. Your lower hand will rise as your abdomen inflates with air. Breathe in slowly through your nose for four counts. Gradually exhale through your mouth for four counts, feeling your abdomen lower. Don't hold your breath. Repeat four or five times.

The First Week after Surgery

Walking. As you know by now, it's important to get out of bed and walk around your room the day after your surgery. It will seem like a daunting task. Gradually increase the length and frequency of your walks as you regain strength.

Breathing. Practice deep breathing with your triflow unit several times a day.

Stretching exercises you can do in bed. Begin performing these mild strengthening exercises while you're in the hospital.

- Reach out with your legs, alternately flexing and pointing your toes. Stretch your arms out in front of your body, as if trying to touch the wall on other side of room. Hold each stretch for 20 to 30 seconds.

- Lying on your back, raise your arm up straight and slowly move it back as if to touch the wall behind you. Move gently as far as you can without pain.

- Raise your arm. Open and close your hand 15 to 20 times, then bend and straighten your elbow. Repeat this three to four times a day.

- Sitting in bed, rotate your shoulders in circular movements, first moving them forward, then down and back.

Exercises after Implant Reconstruction

Your range of movement will increase as your incisions heal and your muscles recover.

ACS exercises. The following seven exercises from the American Cancer Society's booklet *Exercises After Breast Surgery*, are designed to gradually restore your range of motion and strength. These are some suggested exercises. It is important to talk with your doctor prior to starting the exercises so you can decide on a program that is right for you.

It is normal to feel some tightness in your chest and armpit after surgery. The tightness will decrease as you continue your exercise program. It may be helpful to do exercises after a warm shower when your muscles are warm and relaxed (if your doctor has given you permission to shower).

Wear comfortable, loose clothing. Do the exercises until you feel a slow stretch. Hold each stretch at the end of the motion for a count of five. It is normal to feel some pulling as you stretch the skin and muscles that have been shortened because of the surgery.

Do five to seven repetitions of each exercise.

Do all the exercises twice daily until you regain your normal flexibility and strength.

Breathe deeply as you perform each exercise.

The exercises are designed to begin lying down, move to sitting, and then finish standing.

Exercises in lying position. These exercises should be performed on a bed or the floor while lying on your back with knees and hips bent, feet flat.

The Wand Exercise

This exercise helps increase the forward motion of the shoulders. You'll need a broom handle, yardstick, or other similar object to perform this exercise.

- Hold wand in both hands with palms facing up.

- Lift wand up over your head as far as you can, using your unaffected arm to help lift the wand, until you feel a stretch in your affected arm.

- Hold for five seconds.

- Lower arms and repeat five to seven times.

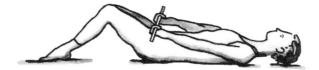

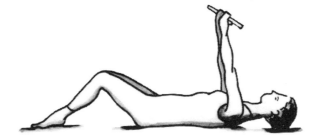

Elbow Winging

This exercise helps to increase the mobility of the front of your chest and shoulder. It may take several weeks of regular exercise before you can get your elbows close to the bed or floor.

- Clasp your hands behind your neck with your elbows pointing toward the ceiling.

- Move your elbows apart and down toward the bed or floor.

- Repeat five to seven times.

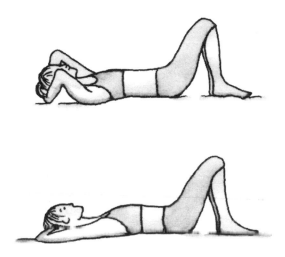

Exercises in Sitting Position. These exercises help increase mobility of the shoulder blade.

Shoulder Blade Stretch

- Sit in a chair very close to a table with your back against the chair back.

- Place uninvolved arm on table with elbow bent and palm down; do not move this arm during the exercise.

- Place affected arm on the table, palm down with elbow straight. Without moving your torso, slide affected arm toward the opposite side of the table. You should feel your shoulder blade move as you do this.

- Relax your arm and repeat five to seven times.

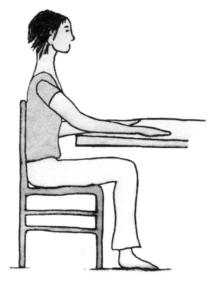

Shoulder Blade Squeeze

- Facing straight ahead, sit in a chair in front of a mirror without resting on the back of the chair.

- Arms should be at your side with elbows bent.

- Squeeze shoulder blades together, bringing your elbows behind you. Keep your shoulders level as you do this exercise. Do not lift your shoulders up toward your ears.

- Return to the starting position and repeat five to seven times.

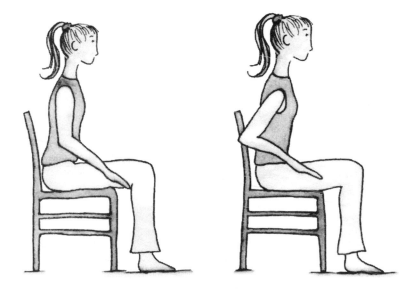

Side Bending

This exercise helps increase mobility of the trunk/body.

- Clasp hands together in front of you and lift your arms slowly over your head, straightening your arms.

- When arms are over your head, bend your trunk to the right while bending at the waist and keeping your arms overhead.

- Return to starting position and bend to the left.

- Repeat the cycle five to seven times.

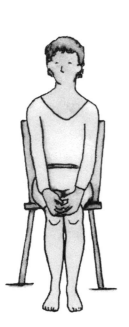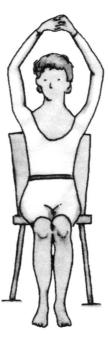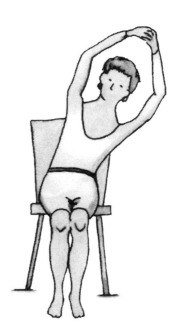

Exercises in Standing Position.

Chest Wall Stretch

This exercise helps stretch the chest wall.

- Stand facing a corner with toes approximately 8 to 10 inches from the corner.

- Bend elbows and place forearms on the wall, one on each side of the corner. Elbows should be as close to shoulder height as possible.

- Keep arms and feet in position and move chest toward the corner.

- You will feel a stretch across your chest and shoulders.

- Return to starting position and repeat five to seven times.

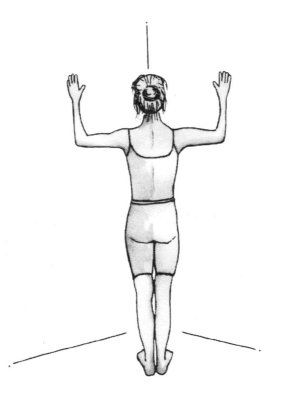

Shoulder Stretch

This exercise helps increase mobility in the shoulder.

- Stand facing the wall with toes approximately 8 to 10 inches from the wall.

- Place your hand on the wall. Use your fingers to "climb the wall," reaching as high as you can until you feel a stretch.

- Return to starting position and repeat five to seven times.

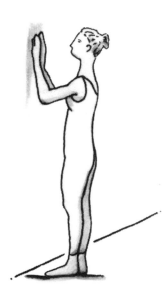
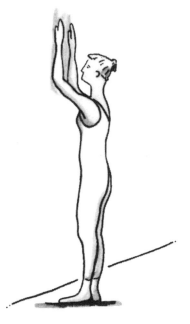

Exercises after Flap Reconstruction

First and second weeks after surgery. Do the exercises described in "The First Week after Surgery."

Third week. Do the exercises described in "Exercises after Implant Reconstruction." If you've had TRAM or DIEP reconstruction, add the following exercises to stretch and strengthen your abdominal muscles.

- Pelvic Tilt. Lie on your back with your knees bent and your feet flat on the floor. Your arms are out to your sides. Gently tighten your abdominal muscles, as if pulling your belly button towards your spine. Hold this position for a count of 10, but don't hold your breath. Release and return to the starting position. Repeat five to 10 times twice each day.

- Trunk stretch. Lie on your back with your knees bent and your feet flat on the floor. Your arms are out to your sides. Slowly let your knees fall to one side, keeping your spine straight and your back flat. Breathe deeply while you hold the pose for a minute or two. Slowly bring your knees back to the starting position and let them fall to the opposite side. Repeat five times twice daily. It may take a few weeks before you can touch your knees to the floor without discomfort.

- Groin stretch. Sit on the floor with your back straight. Place the soles of your feet together. Interlace your fingers around your toes. As much as possible without causing discomfort, lower your knees toward the floor. Repeat three times twice daily.

If you are recovering from a back flap, add the following exercises.

- Butterfly stretch. You can do this exercise with both arms or one arm at a time. Lie flat on the floor or on a flat bench with your arms perpendicular to your body. Bring both arms up above your chest and across towards the opposite shoulder. Repeat 10 times twice daily. At first, you can perform this exercise with your hands empty. As you gain strength, hold soup cans or light dumbbells.

- Back stretch. Lie face down with your chin on the floor. Your arms are stretched out in front of you. Inhale. As you exhale, raise your arms and legs slightly at the same time, with your abdomen touching the floor. Breathe as you hold the pose for 10 seconds. Exhale and lower your arms and legs. Repeat three times twice daily.

Additional Resources

Staying Abreast, written by medical exercise therapist Annie Toglia (a breast cancer survivor with reconstruction), is a comprehensive illustrated exercise program. Eleven rehabilitative workouts are provided to promote recovery from breast surgery, reconstruction, and adjuvant therapies (914-237-1779 or www.stayingabreast.com).

Essential Exercises for Breast Cancer Survivors by Amy Halverstadt and Andrea Leonard provides more than 100 pages of illustrated exercises, divided into four levels of difficulty. Movements to help prevent and manage lymphedema are also included.

Focus on Healing (877-365-6014 or www.focusonhealing.net) is a therapeutic dance-based exercise program designed especially for women after breast cancer surgery. Certified instructors lead a six-week session of low-key exercises designed to increase range of motion, decrease shoulder stiffness, and reduce arm swelling. Based on ballet and jazz dance, the stretching movements can be done by anyone while standing, sitting, or lying in bed. Log on to website to find a class near you, or order the video or book.

The YWCA's Encore Plus is a free post-mastectomy exercise program available to women of all ages and at any stage of the recovery process. Participants exercise on land and in a warm pool (212-273-7800 or contact your local branch). Your local hospital or breast cancer clinic may offer similar classes.

Collage Video features an extensive collection of exercise videotapes, including, strength training, stretching, walking, pilates, yoga, and other activities. (800-433-6769 or www.collagevideo.com). Order online or call for their printed catalog.

Chapter 19

Dealing with Problems

Obstacles don't have to stop you.
If you run into a wall, don't turn around
and give up. Figure out how to climb it,
go through it or work around it.

— Michael Jordan

It's not unusual to encounter aches, pains, spasms, or minor cosmetic imperfections during recovery. Additional procedures may be required to eliminate a dimple in the breast, rebuild a flattened nipple, or remove a pucker of fat. More troublesome problems sometimes occur, as described in the previous chapters about implants and flaps. When problems linger beyond recovery or become severe, corrective steps can and should be taken. The important message here is that you don't have to live with these problems. In most cases, you *can* take action to change what you find unacceptable.

The Best Defense is a Good Offense

While you can't eliminate all possibility of post-recovery complications, you can proactively prevent them from occurring.

Choose an experienced surgeon. Even the best surgeon can't guarantee a problem-free reconstruction. Your own health and the way you heal greatly influence your results. Surgical skill, however, can mean the difference between an acceptable and an unacceptable reconstruction. Choosing a certified, experienced surgeon is perhaps the best single action you can take to guard against post-operative problems.

Manage your expectations. You should have a good understanding of reconstruction by the time you roll into the operating room: how it will be done, how your new breast will look, and what recovery will be like. Knowing what can occur helps you to form realistic expectations. You won't be surprised when your expanding breast sits high on your chest or when it doesn't exactly match the opposite site.

Give yourself adequate time to heal. Many problems and unsatisfactory cosmetic appearances resolve themselves in time. Even though you may acknowledge this intellectually, it's not unusual to hope for instant results. It's easy to feel impatient, but try not to jump to conclusions before you're fully healed. A misshapen or asymmetrical breast may be fine once the swelling disappears and it drops into its final position. It may take a year or more for scars to fade.

Decide what's acceptable and what's not. We are our own harshest critics. Subtle flaws in your breast may be invisible to others, but objectionable to you. It's interesting to note that many women who are somewhat unsatisfied with their reconstructed breasts say their husband or partner thinks it's just fine. One woman may decide she can live with the tiny bulge in her new breast or the wide scar on her tummy. Another may not. After your recovery, you may be unwilling to face yet another procedure, no matter how small. On the other hand, you may want to do anything you can to improve the way your breast looks.

Understand what can be changed; accept what cannot. When all is said and done, some problems cannot be fixed. It's not possible to eliminate scars, for example. Surgeons can't restore full sensation or give you two identical breasts. At some point, you must accept that your reconstruction is as good as it can be, and go on with your life.

Take action. Acknowledging a problem is the first step in treating it. There's no need to suffer in silence. While the thought of additional doctor appointments and procedures may be unsettling, talk to your surgeon about your concerns or dissatisfaction. He's probably seen and heard it all before and can determine whether the problem is likely to run its course or deserves additional attention. If you're unhappy with the way your surgeon handles a post-reconstruction problem, get another opinion. Explain the problem to your insurance company or primary physician and ask for a referral to someone else. Consult a specialist who excels in correcting post-operative problems.

Lingering Pain

There's a very big difference between normal discomfort and chronic or intense pain. While you may decide you can live with cosmetic flaws, you should always seek help for unrelenting pain. Aside from interfering with your well-being, it slows the immune system's ability to fight off disease and infection.

Persistent pain can be caused by a damaged nerve, a hematoma at the mastectomy site, or a variety of other reasons. Sometimes lack of appropriate reconditioning is the cause. A cycle of pain may continue, for example, when you don't properly rehabilitate your arm after surgery: it hurts, you don't use it, it gets worse. Chemotherapy or other adjuvant treatment may contribute to the problem.

Tell your surgeon if you experience excessive pain or strange sensations after reconstruction. He depends on your description to diagnose the probable cause and prescribe an appropriate treatment. Describe the intensity, location, and feeling as accurately as you can. Is it a burning sensation in the nipple? A tingling feeling, a shooting pain, or a dull ache along the outside of the breast? Your surgeon may ask you to log the frequency and severity of your symptoms to help identify the cause.

Post Mastectomy Pain Syndrome. About 30 percent of women develop a burning or tingling in the arm, shoulder, chest wall, or mastectomy scar after axillary lymph node dissection, lumpectomy, or mastectomy. The pain may begin soon after surgery or suddenly appear a year later. It can be continuous or intermittent. This *Post Mastectomy Pain Syndrome* (PMPS) occurs when the *intercostobrachial* nerves that provide sensation to the shoulder and upper arm are severed during surgery. In many cases, the pain can be chronic and debilitating, disrupting sleep and the quality of life.

PMPS is rarely discussed as a potential risk of breast surgery. It is not fully understood or acknowledged by many physicians, who may assume the pain is simply a residual side effect of mastectomy. Talk to your oncologist and surgeon if you develop continuing pain in the area of your mastectomy. If the pain persists, you may need a physical examination and a computerized tomography (CT or CAT) scan—an advanced x-ray technology used to help diagnose problems not visible with traditional x-rays.

PMPS is often treated with oral non-steroidal anti-inflammatory drugs (NSAIDs) or other medicines used to treat nerve pain. Sometimes mild anti-depressants provide relief. Your doctor can also administer a series of nerve-block injections or anesthetic along the nerve path.

Acupuncture, massage, or specialized physical therapy may also control the pain. It may take a process of trial-and-error to find a solution that works for you.

If your pain persists, ask for a referral to a pain clinic or a specialist. In rare cases, there may be no way to repair the damage or eliminate the pain. If this occurs, always get a second opinion, preferably from a doctor who specializes in treatment of PMPS. If the diagnosis remains unchanged, you may have to rely on pain management techniques to control your discomfort.

Lymphedema

Removing lymph nodes can impair the lymph system's ability to drain fluids effectively. When the nodes become clogged, fluid accumulates in the tissues of the arm, causing mild to severe swelling called lymphedema. About 20 percent of women who have nodes removed develop this condition.

My arm, hand, and fingers began to swell right after my mastectomy. I couldn't bend my wrist or straighten my arm all the way, and it throbbed constantly. It was impossible to hold or carry my baby. I suffered for several months until my doctor sent me to a physical therapist. She taught my husband how to do a special massage. We've made this a part of our daily routine. I feel better, and my husband is happy he can do something to help. The lymphedema is still there, but at least it's manageable now. – Skye

There's no way to predict who will get lymphedema and who won't. It may occur soon after breast cancer surgery, or months or years later. The swelling can be almost unnoticeable, like fluid retention during your period. In extreme cases, the arm becomes enlarged from shoulder to fingertips. There is no cure for lymphedema. If treated immediately, however, it can be controlled with compression sleeves, special exercises, and therapeutic massage. Contact your doctor at the first sign of swelling—even mild swelling—in your arm after breast surgery.

Be very protective of your affected arm. Zealously protect it from burns, cuts, and other injuries. Keep it scrupulously clean to avoid infection. Get in the habit of using your opposite arm for lifting, scrubbing, or other vigorous movements. Injections, blood samples, or blood pressure readings should be taken from the unaffected arm as well. Contact the National Lymphedema Network (800-541-3259 or www.lymphnet.org) for more information about preventing and controlling lymphedema. Reach for Recovery, breast cancer organizations, and many hospitals also provide support and information.

Cosmetic Imperfections

It's not uncommon to need a minor operation to improve a newly reconstructed breast, but some fixes are easier than others.

Revision surgery. Cosmetic flaws are often corrected with minor in-patient procedures. A lump of excess skin or a small indentation that mars an otherwise perfect-looking breast can often be corrected when your nipple is created. Complications of larger proportions may require another return to the operating room. If your breast is too big, it can be reduced. If your implant is too small, it can be replaced with a larger device. A breast can be lifted if it's too low or dropped if it's too high. Don't like the position or look of your new nipple? It can be redone.

All these situations can be repaired. The fix may require another operation and a bit more downtime, but to a lesser degree than your initial reconstruction surgery. The worst case scenario is repeating the entire reconstruction. That's when you must consider whether your dissatisfaction outweighs the prospect of all that entails.

Improving Scars

Scarring is a natural part of the body's healing process and an unavoidable side effect of surgery. It is slight when the *epidermis*, or outer layer of skin, is damaged; when you burn your finger or get a paper cut, for example. When the *dermis*, the thick tissue beneath the epidermis, is affected—as when a surgical incision is made—the body produces a connective tissue protein called *collagen* to fill in the gaps. It's the body's version of spackle.

Scars look different than the rest of your skin because collagen looks different. It has no sweat glands or pores. When too much collagen is produced, the result is a thicker, more prominent scar. Why does your friend's TRAM scar look so much better than yours? The appearance of a scar is determined by a person's age, genetics, the depth of the wound, and how the incision and underlying tissues are sewn together. Smoking is also a factor. If you smoke, poor blood flow at the incision site may make your scar more obvious. The scars you have from previous surgeries or wounds are a good indication of how your reconstruction scar will heal.

Reconstruction scars are red and noticeable after surgery. They fade to pink after two to three months, as collagen and new blood vessels heal the incision. Mastectomy and reconstruction scars never disappear, but most fade considerably within a year or two after surgery. Others may remain deeply pigmented, bumpy, or raised.

I couldn't believe how many scars I had after my implant reconstruction. I knew my breast would be scarred, but I wasn't prepared for additional scars from drains, lymph node surgery, and skin grafts. I guess I would do it all again, but it was just kind of a shock.
– Cheryl

What can you do? Here are a few suggestions to promote healing and make your scars smoother, flatter, and less noticeable.

- **Maintain pressure on the wound.** Tightly compressing the edges of your wound after surgery helps to form a thin scar line. Your surgeon will apply a strip of surgical tape to keep the incision from spreading as it heals. Don't remove the tape. He'll do that once the incision has closed and started to heal.

- **Moisturize.** A moist wound heals better than a dry wound. As soon as your incisions close and your surgeon gives you the okay, moisturize your incisions with oil, cream, or lotion containing aloe vera or lanolin. Many women have good results with mineral oil or rose hip oil. Vitamin E oil is also popular, although there's no evidence it improves scar tissue. Alcohol dries the skin; avoid products that list it as one of the first three ingredients. Never moisturize a fresh incision. Applying lotions or creams before the skin is closed encourages infection. That leads to more prominent scarring.

- **Massage the scar line**. As you rub in lotion or cream, massage the scar with your fingertips to stretch and break down fibers under the skin. Apply pressure along the length of the scar, then across it. Massage deeply, but never to the point of pain. Roll the scar between your fingers each day to keep the tissue soft.

- **Protect the area from ultraviolet light**. Your scar may darken and become hard if exposed to sunlight or tanning beds during the first year after surgery. Even indirect sun exposure can have an adverse affect. Always apply a sunblock of SPF 20 or higher with UVA and UVB protection at least 20 minutes before you go outside. Avoid oil-based sun lotions, which actually increase sun damage.

- **Apply a scar management product.** Several over-the-counter scar management products can improve new or older scars. Silicone or hydrogel sheets hydrate and compress scars, improving redness and flattening raised areas. These products must be worn for 12 to 18 hours a day for several months before visible improvement occurs. Ask your surgeon what has worked well for his patients. Many women have had very good results with ScarGuard (877-566-5935 or www.scarguard.com), a quick-drying silicone liquid you brush on twice a day for two to six months. If a more natural solution appeals to you, try a botanical gel, like Mederma (888-925-8989 or www.mederma.com). Other products are available from your surgeon, over the Internet, or at your pharmacy.

Hypertrophic and keloidal scars. Some women develop large, lumpy scars that don't respond to any of the above ministrations. *Hypertrophic* scars rise above the level of the surrounding skin and may remain painful or tender. *Keloids* are hypertrophic scars that spread into the skin around the incision. Although anyone can develop keloids, they are more common in darker-skinned women. If other family members develop keloids, you are more likely to have them as well. Let your surgeon know if you're prone to problem scarring. He can add an extra layer of sutures deep within the tissue. It won't guarantee problem scars won't develop, but it may help.

If all else fails, talk to your surgeon or your dermatologist about the following treatments.

- Cortisone injected at the scar site may reduce collagen production and temporarily soften the tissue.

- NSAIDs commonly used to treat arthritis often improve problem scars. Ask your dermatologist about topical aspirin and other such medications.

If all else fails, your scar can be revised. Your surgeon can cut away the hard scar tissue and re-suture the new incision closed. It's no guarantee your new scar will be better—hypertrophic and keloidal scars recur about half the time—but it may be worth a try if you're dissatisfied. Scar revision can be performed in your surgeon's office under local anesthesia, or when your nipple is created.

My scar had a big pucker right in the front of my breast. In about 20 minutes, my surgeon reopened the incision, cut away the scar tissue, and sewed it back up. It felt tight for a few weeks, and then it healed and looked better than before. – Donna

My mastectomy scar is horrible and thick. My doctor cut around it during my reconstruction, but three years later, it's still pretty bad. I knew that was a possibility; I've never scarred well, even from minor cuts. My doctor said it's as good as it's going to get. – Jean

Chapter 20

Life after Reconstruction

Cancer was a gift that helped me grow.
– Rudolph Giuliani

At last. After months of doctor appointments, tests, surgeries, and recovery, your reconstruction journey is over. Your new breast is in place, and you're ready to move on.

You may feel a wonderful sense of closure as you leave your plastic surgeon's office for the last time. Or you may feel sad or depressed, particularly if you've come to regard him as a trusted friend. This isn't unusual. You've spent a lot of time together during your reconstruction, and now your emotional umbilical cord is about to be severed. Your life is finally getting back to normal.

Back to Work

Returning to work is a giant step on the road back to normal. The workplace can be a positive and caring environment, depending how close you are to your co-workers and how much they know about why you've been away. If, on the other hand, your workplace is a source of stress and uneasiness, take time to consider how you'll deal with it before you return.

Your surgeon will tell you when you've healed enough to return to the job. You may need to ease slowly back into the work routine if the pressures and pace of an entire day are too taxing. Perhaps you can work flex hours or part-time until you're back up to speed. If you still feel fatigued, you may need more time to recuperate. Observe your surgeon's instructions regarding limitations on lifting, stretching, and other movements.

Choosing new paths. Breast cancer gives pause to rethink and reconsider. For many, it creates a desire to recognize and reshuffle priorities. Some women find their previous work no longer matches their post-cancer persona. Many want to become more involved in breast cancer issues, either professionally or on a voluntary basis. If you decide to change jobs or seek a new career, a placement counselor can help you match your passion and skills to new pursuits.

During my recovery, I began to think about what I wanted to do when I was able to work again. Going back to my unsatisfying job wasn't high on my list. I was a changed person and I needed a new start. I left my $55,000-a-year job to begin a daycare center—something I had been contemplating for years.
– Jessie

Dating, Intimacy, and Sex

Whether you're single or married, you may worry about how your reconstructed breast will affect your intimate relationships. Being intimate may be awkward at first. After months of treatment and reconstruction you may feel disconnected from physical pleasure and intimacy. Other factors may also affect how you feel. Chemotherapy or other treatments, for example, can affect your mood, sap your energy, or banish your libido.

Talk with your partner before your reconstruction. Express your feelings and encourage him or her to do the same. Although you're the one who goes through reconstruction and recovery, sharing the experience will make life easier for both of you. Open communication paves the way for you and your partner to be more comfortable with your new breast. Look at your body together. If you're comfortable seeing and touching your reconstructed breast, your partner probably will be too.

Don't feel rejected if your partner doesn't initiate intimacy. He may be afraid to hurt you, or think you're not interested or not ready. A little encouragement goes a long way. Be honest about what is uncomfortable and what isn't until you're fully healed. Your new breast may have limited sensation, but it will still feel like a breast to your partner.

Take your time. You've been through a lot. You may be anxious to get your love life back to normal, or you may need more time to restore your mental, physical, and sexual health. Allow yourself a period of adjustment to get back in the groove. Spend time alone together, just being affectionate and doing the things you love to do. If you feel shy or apprehensive, take it slowly. Suggest hugging, kissing, and cuddling before you progress to the main event. If you feel uneasy when you're undressed, wear lingerie or turn out the lights until you become more comfortable with your new breast. Progress at your own pace. Remember, the brain is the most powerful sexual organ we have. You're still a woman. You're still much more than the sum total of your breasts. If you continue to feel uncomfortable with intimacy, consider joining a support group or seeking professional guidance.

My husband kept ignoring my reconstructed breast. I couldn't feel much there, but emotionally, it was important to me to include it in our lovemaking. When I mentioned this to him he said he was afraid he would hurt me. After we talked about it, we both felt relieved, like a huge barrier between us had been broken down.
– Alma

New relationships. Dating presents an interesting dilemma: when and what do you tell your partner-to-be? "Nice to meet you. My left breast came from my stomach" or "I'm finally getting my nipples done tomorrow!" may be a bit much when you're introduced. The best approach is probably to rely on your gut feeling. Your own comfort with the topic and how you feel about the other person will dictate when you talk about your reconstruction, and how much you say. That might be on your first date when you're getting to know each other, or later in your relationship as you undress.

Follow-Up Care

Whether your breast was removed prophylactically or because of breast cancer, you've reduced your future risk significantly. It's wise to remain vigilant, but you needn't live your life in fear. A lump in your breast after reconstruction might be calcification or pieces of dead tissue. Tell your doctor immediately, so he can determine the cause. A mammogram (if you had flap reconstruction), an ultrasound, or a surgical biopsy may be required to determine the nature of the lump.

Monitor your reconstructed breast. You should examine your own breasts each month and have regular professional examinations as recommended by your oncologist. If a medical professional has never shown you how to correctly do a breast self exam, ask your doctor or nurse to demonstrate. Or listen and watch the instructive online video at the Susan G. Komen Breast Cancer Foundation's website (www.komen.org/bse).

Do your exam at the same time each month. Check both breasts while standing up (in the shower is good) *and* lying down. Look for any redness or swelling. Carefully feel along the chest wall up to the collarbone, across the mastectomy scar, and under the arm for any lumps. Become familiar with the terrain of your new breast. Recognize its lumps and irregularities after surgery, so you can distinguish them from future changes which may occur.

Most women will not need mammograms of their reconstructed breast, because they have almost no remaining breast tissue. If you have a breast reconstructed with an implant, it doesn't need to be screened with a mammogram. You should, however, disclose your implant whenever you're asked about your medical history in the future.

Although few mammography centers are familiar with screening procedures for reconstructed breasts, more doctors are now recommending mammograms after flap reconstruction, particularly for women who are at high risk for recurrence. In two small studies at the University of Michigan, mammograms—or TRAMograms as they are called at the school's medical center—detected cancerous areas in several women who had TRAM flaps.

Recommended Follow-up Care

WHAT	WHO	WHEN
mammogram of healthy breast	qualified technician	annually
manual examination of breast, chest wall, and lymph nodes	you	monthly
	your primary physician or oncologist	every 3 to 6 months for the first 3 years after reconstruction. Every 6 to 12 months during the 4th and 5th years, and annually thereafter.
pelvic exam and PAP smear	your gynecologist	annually (less often if you've had a hysterectomy or an oophorectomy)
select blood tests, depending on the type of breast cancer	your primary physician or oncologist	annually

Your oncologist may also recommend bone scans, X-rays, or other tests.

Source: American Society of Clinical Oncologists and ACS

Monitor the opposite breast. Having annual mammograms is still the best opportunity to catch any future breast cancer at an early stage. If you've had breast cancer in one breast, you are at increased risk—about one percent each year—of developing cancer on the other side, so it's important to continue getting annual mammograms. If your natural breast is augmented, your mammogram must be performed by technicians who are trained to take images of implanted breasts.

Inform your oncologist or primary physician of any of the following conditions, which may be symptoms of recurrence:

- Any change in your breasts.

- Sudden weight loss.

- Persistent abdominal pain.

- Chronic bone pain or tenderness.

- Chest pain or shortness of breath.

- A rash, redness, or swelling that doesn't go away.

- A change in overall health that lasts more than a couple of weeks.

Dealing with Recurrence

Recurrence is unlikely after mastectomy, but sometimes leftover cancer cells form a lump in the skin, the mastectomy scar, or what little breast tissue remains. Some women develop a recurrence in the chest muscle, but that's even more uncommon. A small malignancy in the scar or skin can usually be removed without disturbing the implant or the reconstructed flap. It may also require radiation if you haven't already had it on that side of your chest. Excising a larger tumor may involve removing the implant or part of the flap.

Mending Mind, Body, and Spirit

You've beaten cancer and completed reconstruction. Now what? Now you get on with your life. Undoubtedly, you will be relieved to get back your pre-diagnosis life, before the tests and treatments began. Perhaps, like many breast cancer survivors, you feel a new lease on life. One that compels you to find a fresh balance between physical, emotional, and perhaps spiritual, health.

You may feel the need to take better care of your body, not because anything you did caused your breast cancer, but because living with the disease gives us such a profound gratitude for the bodies we have.

For some, it's cause to reassess or reaffirm beliefs. Perhaps you have renewed conviction to travel, change jobs, help others, or do all those things you've always wanted to do, but put on the back burner when life got in the way.

You'll probably never forget your breast cancer. And maybe that's a good thing, because we all learn important lessons from our cancer experiences. Most of us can't simply flick an emotional switch and go seamlessly from patients to disease-free women. It takes time and effort. It's good to look back and reflect. It's better to look forward and embrace the future.

In that wonderful movie, "As Good As It Gets," Helen Hunt's character tells Jack Nicholson's character to give her a compliment, a really good compliment. Nicholson thinks for a while, and then says, "You make me want to be a better man." That's the effect breast cancer often has on women; it makes them want to take better care of themselves, be better people, and to live better lives.

Your Turn to Share

If you're inclined to share what you've learned from your breast cancer experience, lots of women facing mastectomy want to know more about breast cancer treatment and reconstruction. Whether you spend an occasional hour or get involved full-time, there are plenty of opportunities to donate your time, money, and insight.

- Let your oncologist and plastic surgeon know you will be happy to speak with other patients who have questions. Many women will welcome your insight as they consider their post-mastectomy choices and wonder what reconstruction is like.

- Call the ACS to become a Reach to Recovery volunteer.

- Speak to women in your local breast cancer center or support group.

- Donate or raise money for your local breast cancer organization. There are hundreds, if not thousands of local fundraisers for breast cancer each year across the country. There's Sing for the Cure, Run for the Cure, Crop for the Cure, Cruise for the Cure, Art for the Cure, and many more worthwhile efforts. Call your local ACS office or search the internet for "breast cancer charity" to find ways to make a difference.

Chapter 21

Searching for Silver Bullets

Research is the art of seeing what everyone else has seen, and doing what no one else has done.

– Anonymous

One day, this book will be obsolete. Doctors will have tools to prevent breast cancer or at least treat it without removing the breast. Perhaps they'll prescribe an effective antidote or manipulate a patient's genes to turn the disease off. We'll look back on the era of mastectomy and think how archaic that treatment was.

Billions of dollars and countless hours of research by dedicated professionals translate into dramatic improvements. We can now detect breast cancer earlier, treat it more effectively, and produce near-natural reconstruction. Deaths from breast cancer are steadily declining. We've learned much about the disease in the past decade, but we still have a long way to go to find the answers we need. The process isn't easy, and it isn't quick. Some research paths turn out to be dead ends. Practical application is preceded by years of clinical testing and government approval. But we're on the right track, and several exciting advancements are under study or already making their way into the medical mainstream.

Tracking progress. The Internet makes easy work of staying current with research developments. Visit any of the following websites for the latest in breast cancer detection, treatment, and reconstruction.

www.webmd.com

www.medscape.com

www.komen.org

www.susanlovemd.com

www.breast-cancer-research.com

www.cancer.gov/clinicaltrials/breast-cancer-updates

Redefining Early Detection

Today, early detection means finding cancer before it spreads beyond the breast. That's certainly desirable, but we must do more. While mammography is still our best tool for early detection, it's far from perfect, frequently resulting in false positives and undetected tumors. MRI and ultrasound can pinpoint tumors but are too expensive to be used routinely. Researchers are now thinking out of the box, looking for ways to identify potentially dangerous cells before they become cancerous.

Breast cancer blood test. We already have blood tests to find prostate cancer and bladder cancer. Now scientists have identified *nuclear matrix protein-66*, a protein that triggers growth of invasive cancers and some that are non-invasive. If a blood test can be developed to accurately identify the protein, it may replace surgical biopsy as a method of clarifying questionable or suspicious mammogram images.

Positron Emission Tomography (PET). PET scans often identify cancers not detected by other imaging methods. Used to study the brains of stroke victims and the nervous systems of epileptic patients, PET scans can also detect breast cancer. Patients are first given a small amount of radioactive glucose. The scan highlights cancerous tissue, which absorbs more glucose than the rest of the body. Because PET scans are expensive and not always covered by insurance, they used primarily to detect breast cancer in women for whom mammography is less effective, including women who have:

- Breast implants.

- Very dense breast tissue.

- A lump at the mastectomy site.

- A large mass that can be felt but doesn't show up clearly on mammogram or ultrasound.

Enhanced Genetics

Genetic testing and manipulation hold the key to predicting and preventing breast cancer. Although genetics is a new technology, scientists are learning more each year about the relationship of gene defects and breast cancer.

The swab test. Current testing for BRCA1/2 gene mutations requires a blood sample and can cost up to $2,800 per patient. Researchers at Bay State Medical Center in Springfield, Mass., believe they've found an easier, less expensive method. They've discovered gene mutations slightly change a particular protein in the body. Swabbing a few cells from a patient's mouth may be enough to determine if the protein is present.

The DBC2 gene. In 2002, researchers made another important genetic discovery. They identified the DBC2 ("Deleted in Breast Cancer") gene and a protein that controls abnormal cell growth. When the gene is missing or not working properly, a woman is more likely to develop breast cancer. This may be a milestone discovery; defective or missing DBC2 genes may cause up to 60 percent of non-hereditary breast cancers. In one small study, tumors stopped growing when they were injected with healthy DBC2 genes. In the future, we may prevent breast cancer by replacing or repairing these genes.

Estrogen-cellular relationship. In 2003, German researchers discovered how estrogen is monitored at the cellular level. This knowledge may ultimately provide a way to stop estrogen-positive breast cancer cells from multiplying.

Kinder, Gentler Biopsies

More than a million women have surgical breast biopsies each year—procedures that find cancer in only 10 to 15 percent of patients, yet scar each and every one. While biopsies are minor procedures, they cause a great deal of patient anxiety and cost the U.S. health care system an estimated $2.3 billion.

From a reconstructive perspective, a surgical biopsy leaves a scar that remains on the new breast. In many cases, the following less invasive procedures can be performed in an hour or less without scarring.

Advanced Breast Biopsy Instrumentation (ABBI). During this computer-guided procedure, the patient lies with her breast dangling through a hole in a special table. Using ultrasound to first pinpoint the exact location of the tumor, a physician inserts a thin needle into the breast and extracts a small tissue sample for examination by a pathologist.

Mammotone biopsy. A *Mammotone biopsy* is similar to the ABBI technique, except most or all of the questionable tissue is suctioned from the breast with a special needle. Patients sometimes develop a bruise or a hematoma where the needle is inserted, but the procedure has no serious side effects. Women whose lesions are close to an implant, next to chest wall muscles, or less than 1.5 cm may be candidates for this less invasive procedure.

Ductal lavage. By painlessly extracting fluid from the milk ducts, doctors can identify pre-cancerous cells long before a mammogram can find them—up to 10 years before a tumor forms. This ductal lavage, called the Pap smear for the breast, is currently in limited use as a diagnostic for high-risk women. When atypical breast cells are found, patients may choose preventative actions before breast cancer develops, including:

- Taking tamoxifen for its preventative properties.

- Monitoring their breasts more frequently with physical exams, MRI, and ultrasound.

- Considering prophylactic mastectomy (if they have BRCA1/2 gene mutations or a family history of breast cancer).

Lavage is relatively inexpensive and easy to learn. In the future, it may become a routine screening procedure for all women. Contact ProDuct Health (866-446-3828 or www.producthealth.com) for more information or to find a physician who performs ductal lavage.

Ductoscopy. Another non-invasive method of detecting precancerous cells involves *ductoscopy*. By inserting an ultra-thin, fiberoptic magnifying scope through the nipple, surgeons can see directly into the ducts and remove cellular samples without surgery. Potential candidates for the procedure include women who:

- Have discharge from the nipple.

- Have questionable mammograms.

- Have had multiple biopsies.

- Have a strong family history of breast or ovarian cancer.

- Are taking hormone replacement therapy.

Laser imaging. At Clemson University, a preliminary laser technology called *optical tomographic imaging* produces a three-dimensional image of the breast. Because cancerous tissues absorb laser light differently than normal tissue, laser imaging holds promise for distinguishing between benign and malignant tumors.

MR elastography. Current magnetic resonance imaging (MRI) technology can detect some breast cancers, but produces many false positives. Mayo Clinic researchers are developing *MR elastography,* a new method of combining MRI with sound waves to measure the elasticity of breast tissue tumors. This new process detects malignant tumors, which tend to be harder and less elastic than healthy breast tissue.

Innovative Treatments

New tools in the fight against breast cancer allow doctors to refine and individualize treatments.

Molecular profiling. Current treatments for breast cancer are standardized. Generally, similar regimens are recommended for women with tumors of the same type and size. We know this standardized approach is too aggressive for some patients and too conservative for others, but for now, it's our best remedy. Our growing knowledge of DNA, however, is reshaping the future of treatment. *Molecular profiling* identifies specific protein patterns in blood or tissue. It's a process that can help predict how an individual's breast cancer will grow. Treatments can then be customized accordingly.

Radiation after lumpectomy. Traditional radiation delivered from outside the body destroys cancer cells, but also damages healthy tissue and skin. The next generation of radiation involves delivery from the inside out, targeting only the area around the tumor. Newer methods of radiation could benefit the 70 percent of breast cancer patients with early-stage tumors.

- Standard post-lumpectomy radiation includes daily treatment for five to eight weeks. A five-year study at Hamilton Regional Cancer Center in Canada suggests three weeks of radiation is just as effective. Rates of recurrence were the same—about three percent—in the study group of 1,200 women. Some patients on the shortened schedule received higher daily doses of radiation than those with longer treatment schedules.

- Studies are underway to determine whether a single, short dose of radiation delivered while the patient is still on the operating table is as effective as the current five-to-eight-week treatment.

- *Brachytherapy,* the same radiation therapy used to treat prostate cancer, involves placing several thin catheters in the breast around the tumor site. This can be done while the patient is still on the operating table or during a later procedure. The patient returns to the radiation facility twice daily for five days. Radioactive material is placed in each of the catheters for five to 15 minutes, and then withdrawn. After the final application, the catheters are removed. Radiation is delivered precisely to the tumor site without affecting healthy tissue or skin. The entire treatment is completed in just five days. A variation of brachytherapy places a small balloon at the tumor site after lumpectomy. A single catheter runs from the balloon to the outside of the breast, through which radiation seeds are delivered twice daily for five days. The balloon is then deflated and the catheter is removed.

Destroying tumors with radio waves. Breakthrough treatments for other cancers may also hold promise. Doctors at the M.D. Anderson Cancer Center are using high-frequency radio waves to vaporize breast cancer tumors without damaging surrounding healthy tissue. Clinical tests have been completed, and the procedure is awaiting FDA approval.

Breast cancer vaccine. We may be closing in on the magic pill, or injection, as it were. Using a newly developed vaccine, researchers can stop breast cancer from developing in mice. Hopefully, a preventative vaccine for humans isn't far behind. Vaccines can also be used to treat disease. Trials of Theratope, a serum for women with advanced breast cancer, are underway with 1,030 patients in 10 countries. Results should be available near the end of 2003. The vaccine, which appears to have few side effects, stimulates a patient's own immune system to attack and destroy cancerous cells. Contact Biomira (780-450-3761 or www.biomira.com) for more information.

Pioneering Reconstructive Techniques

Growing new breasts. If a woman's body could be prompted to grow a new breast, we could eliminate the cost, time, angst, scarring, and discomfort inherent with reconstruction. Tissue engineering, or stem cell research, may be the answer. Found in bone marrow, blood, and embryos, stem cells are the body's building blocks. They are genetic blank slates, awaiting orders to evolve into bone, lungs, heart, or any kind of tissue the body needs.

Researchers believe stem cells are the key to the body's self-repair—if we learn how to nudge the cells in certain directions, we can repair physical defects at the cellular level. The therapy is already used to replace leukemia patients' cells that are damaged or destroyed by chemotherapy. Solving the mystery of stem cells could put an end to diseases now considered incurable. The possibilities are endless. If we can generate new tissue and bone, people with paralyzing spinal cord injuries might walk again. Transplants could become a thing of the past. Need a kidney? Doctors will grow one for you. Eyesight failing? Perhaps a stem cell infusion will create new, improved vision. Women's post-mastectomy choices could include breast regrowth instead of breast reconstruction.

As far-fetched as this seems, researchers at the Bernard O'Brien Institute of Microbiology in Melbourne, Australia, have already grown a breast-shaped blob of fat on a rabbit's groin and transplanted it to the animal's chest. The process involves stimulating stem cells to create fatty tissue, which grows within the confines of an implanted breast-shaped gel infrastructure. (Growing breast tissue is possible, but carries the risk of breast cancer, so fatty tissue, which makes up most of a healthy breast, was grown instead.) The next step in the research process is figuring out how to control tissue growth—how to turn it off once the new breast grows to a desired size, for example.

Sparing the nipple. Mastectomy typically involves removing as much breast tissue as possible, including the nipple and areola. Increasingly, women facing mastectomy and reconstruction want their nipples saved to retain sensation. Although most doctors agree nipple-sparing is emotionally important for patients, they're concerned about potentially increasing the risk of recurrence. Plastic surgeons at M.D. Anderson Cancer Center and Memorial Sloan-Kettering Cancer Center are studying rates of recurrence, and under what, if any, circumstances nipple-sparing might be appropriate. While it will certainly be unwise for many patients, it could be an option for some mastectomy patients, including:

- Women whose cancer does not involve the nipple.

- Women with early-stage non-invasive cancer confined to the ducts or lobules.

- Women who remove their breasts prophylactically.

Restoring sensation. Many women are satisfied with their reconstructed breasts except for the loss of feeling. Some sensation is regained as nerves regenerate. Additional feeling can be restored if the intercostal nerve in a tissue flap is connected to a nerve at the mastectomy site. Most fine sensation in the breast, however, is lost permanently. Surgeons at Johns Hopkins Center for Aesthetic and Reconstructive Surgery of the Breast are studying whether nerves from a tissue flap can be successfully transplanted in the reconstructed breast. This will require greater microsurgical qualifications and skills, but may one day become a standard feature of flap reconstruction.

Someday...

...we'll put breast cancer where it belongs: alongside polio, small pox, and whooping cough on the list of diseases we've cured and no longer fear.

Glossary

Adjuvant therapy Treatment given after surgery.

Areola The dark area around the nipple.

Attached flap A portion of skin, fat and muscle used to recreate a new breast, and which remains tethered to its original blood supply.

Autologous flap Skin, fat and muscle taken from somewhere on a woman's body to form a breast.

Axillary node dissection Surgical removal of underarm lymph nodes to determine whether cancer has spread beyond the breast.

Back flap Skin, fat and muscle taken from the back to form a breast.

Bilateral mastectomy Surgical removal of both breasts.

Bilateral reconstruction Recreation of both breasts after mastectomy.

Biopsy Removing tissue to determine whether cancer cells are present.

BRCA1 (BReast CAncer gene 1) A gene which, when muta increases the risk of developing breast and ovarian cancers.

BRCA2 (BReast CAncer gene 2) A gene which, when muta increases the risk of developing breast and ovarian cancers.

Breast augmentation Surgically enlarging the breast with an imp

Breast cancer Cancer that starts in the breast.

Breast form An artificial breast that can be worn after mastector provide a natural profile in clothing.

Breast implant A rubberized sac filled with saline or silicone gel that is surgically implanted to increase breast size or restore breast shape after mastectomy.

Breast lift A surgical procedure to position sagging breasts higher on the chest.

Breast mound A reconstructed breast without a nipple or areola.

Breast reconstruction Surgery using an implant or a patient's own tissue to rebuild her breast after mastectomy.

Breast reduction Surgery to reduce the size of the breast.

Capsular contracture Squeezing or distortion of an implant caused by a capsule of hard scar tissue.

Chemotherapy A drug treatment used to destroy cancer cells.

Delayed reconstruction Creating a new breast after a woman has recovered from mastectomy.

DIEP flap Abdominal skin and fat used to recreate a breast. No muscle is used.

Donor site The place on the body where tissue is borrowed to recreate a breast.

Duct The part of the breast that delivers milk to the nipple.

Ductal lavage A non-surgical breast biopsy technique.

Exchange surgery A secondary reconstructive surgery to exchange a tissue expander for an implant.

Flap An island of skin, fat, tissue and sometimes muscle, moved from somewhere on the body to the chest to reconstruct a breast.

Free flap A flap that is completely removed from the donor site and transplanted to the chest.

Genetic Related to the genes.

Genetic counselor A specially-trained professional who can calculate a woman's risk of developing breast cancer.

Genetic mutations Changes in the genes that may cause cancer.

Genetics The study of genes.

Genetic testing Laboratory examination of a person's blood to determine whether genetic mutations occur.

Gluteal flap Skin, fat and muscle from the buttocks used to create a breast.

Hematoma A collection of blood at the incision site.

Hereditary breast cancer A cancer which is passed from parent to child.

Immediate reconstruction Recreating a new breast while the patient is still asleep from the mastectomy procedure.

Invasive breast cancer Breast cancer that can spread beyond the breast to other parts of the body.

Latissimus dorsi flap A type of reconstruction that uses the flat muscle in the back to recreate the breast.

Lobule The milk-producing gland in the breast.

Lumpectomy Surgery to remove a breast tumor and a small amount of surrounding tissue.

Lymph nodes Small bean-shaped glands that defend the body from bacteria.

Lymph node biopsy Surgical removal of some or all underarm lymph nodes to determine whether cancer cells have spread from the breast.

Lymph system A part of the immune system that filters body waste.

Lymphedema Mild to severe swelling from the hand to the shoulder that may occur after lymph nodes are removed or the breast is irradiated.

Mammogram An x-ray used to determine whether breast cancer is present in the breast.

Mammoplasty Surgical augmentation or reduction of the breast.

Mastectomy Surgical removal of the breast.

Mastopexy Surgery to reposition the breast so it is higher on the chest.

Microsurgeon A medical professional who is trained to use a surgical microscope to perform very intricate surgery, such as dissecting and reconnecting blood vessels.

Modified radical mastectomy Removal of the entire breast, nipple, areola, and often the underarm lymph nodes.

Necrosis Tissue death from insufficient blood supply.

Needle biopsy A non-surgical sample of breast cells removed with a needle.

Neoadjuvant therapies Treatment given before surgery.

Non-invasive breast cancer Breast cancer that is incapable of spreading beyond the breast.

Oncologist A medical professional who specializes in the treatment of cancer.

Oophorectomy Surgical removal of the ovaries.

Pathologist A medical professional who examines cells to determine if cancerous cells are present.

Pedicled flap A portion of skin, fat and muscle used to recreate a new breast, and remains tethered to its original blood supply. Same as an attached flap.

Plastic surgeon A specially-trained medical professional who specializes in cosmetic or reconstructive surgery.

Prophylactic mastectomy Surgical removal of the breast to reduce the risk of developing breast cancer.

Prosthesis An artificial breast worn after mastectomy to provide a natural profile in clothing. Same as breast form.

Ptosis Drooping of the breasts.

Quadrantectomy Surgery to remove a breast tumor and a large portion (often a quarter) of the surrounding tissue.

Radiation High-energy waves used to destroy cancer cells and prevent recurrence.

Radical mastectomy Removal of the entire breast, nipple, areola, pectoral muscles, and lymph nodes. This procedure is rarely performed today.

Revision surgery A surgical procedure performed to improve the results of an earlier cosmetic or reconstructive surgery.

Risk factor Something that influences whether a person does or doesn't develop cancer.

Saline A saltwater solution used to fill expanders and some implants.

Scar A permanent change in the texture of the skin after it heals from a burn, cut or other injury.

Sentinel node biopsy A minimally invasive method of sampling lymph nodes to determine whether cancer has spread beyond the breast.

Seroma A collection of fluid at the incision site.

Silicone A manmade material used to fill some implants. It is also used for the outer shells of all implants.

Simple mastectomy Removal of the breast, skin and nipple. Lymph nodes are not removed. Same as a total mastectomy.

Skin graft A portion of skin which is moved from one part of the body to the other, such as using a skin graft from the hip to create an areola.

Skin-sparing mastectomy A mastectomy performed to preserve most of the breast skin to facilitate immediate reconstruction.

Surgical drain A plastic bulb that collects fluids at the incision site after surgery.

Symmetry The physical and aesthetic balance between a woman's breasts.

Tattoo A method of applying pigment to a reconstructed nipple and areola.

Thigh flap Skin, fat and muscle taken from the thigh to reconstruct a breast.

Tissue expander A temporary saline implant used to stretch the skin sufficiently to make room for a fixed-volume implant.

Total mastectomy. Removal of the breast, skin and nipple. Lymph nodes are not removed. Same as a simple mastectomy.

TRAM flap Skin, fat and muscle taken from the abdomen to reconstruct a breast.

Unilateral mastectomy Surgical removal of one breast.

Unilateral reconstruction Recreation of one breast after mastectomy.

Resources

Organizations

American Cancer Society
800-227-2345 or www.cancer.org

Living Beyond Breast Cancer
610-645-4567 or www.lbbc.org

National Alliance of Breast Cancer Organizations
888-806-2226 or www.nabco.org

National Cancer Institute
800-422-6237 or www.cancer.gov

National Lymphedema Network
800-541-3259 or www.lymphnet.org

Reach to Recovery
800-227-2345 or www.cancer.org

Susan G. Komen Breast Cancer Foundation
800-462-9273 or www.komen.org

Susan Love, MD Breast Cancer Foundation
805-963-2877 or www.susanlovemd.com

Y-ME National Breast Cancer Organization
800-221-2141 or www.y-me.org

Breast Cancer Genetics and Risk

Assess Your True Risk of Breast Cancer by Patricia T. Kelly, Ph.D.
(www.ptkelly.com)

Facing Our Risk of Cancer Empowered (FORCE)
www.facingourrisk.org

Myriad Genetics
800-725-2722 or www.myriad.com

National Society of Genetic Counselors
610-872-7608 or www.nsgc.org

Coping

The Cancer Club
800-586-9062 or www.cancerclub.com

Kids Konnected
800-899-2866 or www.kidskonnected.org

Kidscope
404-233-0002 or www.kidscope.org

The Well Spouse Foundation
800-838-0879 or www.wellspouse.org

Exercise

Exercises after Breast Surgery, ACS
800-227-2345 or www.cancer.org

Staying Abreast
914-237-1779 or www.stayingabreast.com

Yoga and the Gentle Art of Healing: A Journey of Recovery after Breast Cancer (video)
858-481-3912 or www.yogajoyofdelmar.com

YWCA Encore Plus Program
800-953-7587 or www.ywca.org

Health Insurance

Dept. of Labor, Pensions and Welfare Benefits Admin.
800-998-7542 or www.askebsa.dol.gov

National Insurance Consumer Helpline
800-942-4242 or www.iii.org

Implants and Tissue Flaps

Breast Reconstruction: What You Need to Know (CD-ROM)
M.D. Anderson Cancer Center
713-794-1247 or www.mdanderson.org/breastreconstruction

Federal Drug Administration (FDA)
888-463-6332 or www.fda.gov/cdrh/breastimplants

Information for Women about the Safety of Silicone Breast Implants
by the Institute of Medicine
Y-ME National Breast Cancer Organization
800-221-2141 or www.y-me.org

Making an Informed Decision
Inamed Aesthetics
800-862-4426 or www.inamed.com

Mentor Corporation
800-525-0245 or www.mentorcorp.com

Bibliography

Books/Pamphlets

American Cancer Society, Inc. *Exercises after Breast Surgery*, 2001 and *Mastectomy: A Patient Guide*, 1997.

Berger, Karen and Bostwick, John, *A Woman's Decision: Breast Care, Treatment and Reconstruction*, St. Martin's Griffin, New York, 1998.

Food and Drug Administration. *Breast Implants: an Information Update*, 2000.

Kelly, Patricia, *Assess Your True Risk of Breast Cancer*, Henry Holt and Company, New York, 2000.

Love, Susan M., with Karen Lindsey, *Dr. Susan Love's Breast Book*, Perseus Publishing, Cambridge, 2000.

Rosenthal, Sara M., *The Breast Sourcebook*, Lowell House, Los Angeles, 1999.

Weiss, Ellen and Weiss, Marisa, *Living Beyond Breast Cancer*, Times Books, 1998.

Publications

Chen, PY. Brachytherapy zaps breast cancer. Study presented to the American Society for Therapeutic Radiology and Oncology annual meeting 2002.

Collins, DE, et al. Surgical treatment of early breast cancer: what would surgeons choose for themselves? Effective Clinical Practice 1999; 2:149-151.

Diana, M. Nipple-areola reconstruction. *eMedicine Journal* 2001.

Evans, GR, et al: Reconstruction and the radiated breast: is there a role for implants? 48th Cancer Symposium of the Society of Surgical Oncologists 1995.

Gorman, C. Rethinking breast cancer. *Time* 2002.

Hamaguchi, M, et al. DBC2, a candidate for a tumor suppressor gene involved in breast cancer. *The Proceedings* 2002; 13647-13652.

John, L. Mastectomy update: the good, the bad and the beautiful. *Breast Cancer Action Newsletter* 1998.

Kauff, ND, et al. Risk-reducing Salpingo-oophorectomy in women with a BRCA1 or BRCA2 mutation. *The New England Journal of Medicine* 2002; 346:1609-1615.

Laino, C. Sprouting new breast tissue. MSNBC 2002

Lebovic, GS, et al. Aesthetic approach to simple and modified radical mastectomy. *Contemporary Surgery* 1994; 45:15-19.

Metcalfe, KA and Narod, SA. Breast cancer risk perception among women who have undergone prophylactic bilateral mastectomy. *Journal of the National Cancer Institute* 2002; 20:1564-1569

Moran, SL and Serletti, JM. Outcome comparison between free and pedicled TRAM flap bresat reconstruction in the obese patient. *Reconstructive Surgery* 2001; 108:1954-1960.

Nahabedian, M. Breast reconstruction with expanders and implants: choosing between the 1-stage and 2-stage techniques. *Artemis* 2002.

Padubidri, AN, Yetman, R, et al. Complications of postmastectomy breast reconstruction in smokers, ex-smokers, and nonsmokers. *Plastic & Reconstructive Surgery* 2001; 107:342-349.

Rogers, NE and Allen, RJ. Radiation effects on breast reconstruction with the deep inferior epigastric perforator flap. *Plastic & Reconstructive Surgery* 2002; 109:1919-1924.

Singletary, SE. Skin-sparing mastectomy with immediate breast reconstruction. Is it safe? *Breast Diseases* 1995. 6:259-260.

Tran, NV, et al. Postoperative adjuvant irradiation: effects on transverse rectus abdominis muscle flap breast reconstruction. *Plastic Reconstructive Surgery* 2000; 1:106(2); 313-7.

Wanzel, KR, et al. Reconstructive breast surgery: referring physician knowledge and learning needs. *Plastic and Reconstructive Surgery* 2002; 110(6):1441-1450.

Wilkins, E. Michigan breast reconstruction outcome study 2000.

Yano, K, Mastsuo, Y, and Hosokawa, K. Breast reconstruction by means of innervated rectus abdominis myocutaneous flap. *Plastic & Reconstructive Surgery* 1998; 02:1452-1460.

Index

Give the Gift of Information

To order:

Call: 1-800-431-1579   Online: www.breastrecon.com

Fax: 1-650-592-3790   E-mail: carlop@pacbell.net

US mail: Carlo Press, PO Box 7019, San Carlos, CA 94070

Yes, I want ___ copies of *The Breast Reconstruction Guidebook* at $19.95 each plus $4.00 shipping and handling per book. (CA residents please add $1.65 sales tax)

My check or money order for $_____.___ is enclosed.

Please charge my credit card:

□ Mastercard   □ Visa   □ Amex   □ Discover

Card # _____Exp. Date _____

Signature_____

Name _____

Address_____

City/State/Zip_____

Phone _____ E-mail_____

Our other publications:

The Scrapbooker's Guide to Business:
What You Need to Know Before You Invest
Wondering how you can turn your scrapbooking passion into a profitable business? Find what you need to get started in nine different part-time and full-time business. $14.95

Meals and Memories: How to Create Keepsake Cookbooks
A comprehensive guide for preserving family recipes and treasured memories. $15.95

All books are shipped USPS Priority Mail.